The Teen
Weight-Loss
Solution

ALSO BY ERIKA SCHWARTZ, M.D.

Natural Energy
The Hormone Solution
The 30-Day Natural Hormone Plan

The Teen Weight-Loss Solution

The Safe and Effective Path to

Health and Self-Confidence

ERIKA SCHWARTZ, M.D.

WILLIAM MORROW

An Imprint of HarperCollins*Publishers*

This book contains advice and information relating to health care. It is not intended to replace medical advice and should be used to supplement rather than replace regular care by your doctor. It is recommended that you seek your physician's advice before embarking on any medical program or treatment. All efforts have been made to ensure the accuracy of the information contained in this book as of the date of publication. The publisher and the author disclaim liability for any medical outcomes that may occur as a result of applying the methods suggested in this book.

FIRST EDITION

Designed by Mia Risberg

Printed on acid-free paper

Library of Congress Cataloging-in-Publication Data

Schwartz, Erika.
    The teen weight-loss solution: the safe and effective path to health and self-confidence / Erika Schwartz.—1st ed.
        p. cm.
    Includes bibliographical references.
    ISBN 0-06-073932-0
        1. Obesity in adolescence. 2. Weight loss. 3. Teenagers—Nutrition. 4. Reducing diets. I. Title.

RJ399.C6S39 2004
613.2'5'08352—dc22   2004042682

04 05 06 07 08 WBC/QW 10 9 8 7 6 5 4 3 2 1

To Rachel Wachtel—
to your beauty, your sweetness,
and your future

Contents

Acknowledgments

Deborah Schneider, my agent and great friend: I thank you for always believing in me and leading me to the great Claire Wachtel. The journey certainly was worth the time!

Thank you, Claire Wachtel. You changed my life. You brought me Rachel, who I fell in love with from the first time I saw her. You brought me to William Morrow and introduced me to a great group of people I love working with. You made the process fun and exciting! Thank you to Michael Morrison and my new family at Morrow/HarperCollins. I never thought I'd write a book working in a corporate office. You helped me do it, welcomed me, and encouraged me every step of the way.

To Eve Krzyzanowski, thank you for your commitment, your enthusiasm, and your good advice.

To all my patients who have brought me their daughters and helped me understand teenagers, thank you!

To my daughters, Lisa and Katie, thank you for choosing me as your mother, keeping me involved in your lives, and trusting me. You are wonderful young women! Life with you is pure joy and the most important part of my world!

To my husband, Ken, thank you for your unwavering support and love. It is fully and freely reciprocated.

To Bethany, Ben, and Katie, thank you for your trust and kindness. You are remarkable, and the future is yours!

Introduction

Teenage obesity and diabetes have reached epidemic proportions in the United States.

As adults get fatter, so too do our teens.

Along with this epidemic increase in obesity comes a raft of health problems previously associated with older Americans—heart disease, infertility, mental sluggishness, and hormone imbalances.

Our children, already addicted to such sedentary pursuits as television and the Internet and raised on a diet of junk food, are now obese, unhappy, and hormonally challenged.

On December 2, 2003, the *New York Times* wrote: "We no longer have to wait until age 40 for the first heart attack or the start of diabetes. The way our teens are living, they are at risk now."

In 2001 *Newsweek* noted that our girls are now entering puberty earlier. "The suspected culprits appear to include increased body fat content and eating foods treated with synthetic hormones."

In January 2004, *Newsweek* addressed the top ten health problems of 2003. Number one was obesity, with kids and teens joining the adult ranks in frightening and rapidly growing numbers.

The future doesn't look promising. As the mother of a preteen or teenager, you want to know what to do. She is getting fat, has low self-esteem, is miserable, and has a face covered with pimples. You can no longer communicate, she hates you, and just looking at her breaks your heart.

Is this teen disaster something you need to learn to live with and hope your child survives it?

Is there hope?

The answer is yes! There is hope, and I have the plan you should follow. *The Teen Weight-Loss Solution* is the result of my experience of over twenty-seven years in clinical practice, more than fifty thousand patients cared for, ten years of expertise in balancing hormones, and more than five hundred teens successfully carried to adulthood.

I am the mother of two girls, ages twenty-six and nineteen. Raising them successfully is my best credential. I will share with you what I did right and what I did wrong. Raising teens is not a clinical endeavor—it is a human accomplishment.

By the time you have read this book, you will have become the expert on your teen.

The Teen Weight-Loss Solution follows many personal stories. They come from my patients, my children, and their friends.

This is not a dry treatise on adolescent woes. It is a personalized, easy-to-understand prescriptive on how you and your child can happily and healthily survive the teenage years. They need not be traumatic.

The trip to a healthy life and protection from disease and aging starts now.

How Do You Know If Your Teen Is Overweight?

Before I give you a detailed explanation of what your nutritionist, physician, and high school nurse are using as criteria for defining whether your teen is overweight, I want to help by introducing common sense in your determination of your teen's weight status.

You know your teen better than anyone else. You have watched her grow from a little baby into a young woman. You don't need a degree in nutrition to look at your child and figure out if she has a weight problem. If she does have a problem, you may then need help quantifying it. That is when you need the definitions and criteria that follow.

COMMONSENSE DEFINITIONS OF OVERWEIGHT AND OBESITY

Here are a few guidelines, stemming from my professional experience and common sense, that I believe you will find helpful in determining your teen's weight status and a lot less intimidating than the medical definitions with their scary implications.

Your teen is overweight if:

- Her clothes size increases even though she is not getting taller or increasing her muscle mass through increased physical activity.
- You notice (without being overly critical) that she has developed love handles that hang over her clothes.

- Her belly protrudes and you can see a couple of rolls through her sweater, even though she wears larger sweaters and T-shirts and keeps pulling them down.
- She wears increasingly larger and bulkier clothes to cover up her growing girth.
- Her wrists and ankles are growing in size without increases in the size of her hands and feet.
- She is developing a double chin, and no one else in the family had a double chin at her age.
- Her rear end is increasing in size along with her thighs, and she is developing cellulite.

Bear these commonsense guidelines in mind as you review the more technical definitions that follow.

MEDICAL DEFINITIONS
OF OVERWEIGHT AND OBESITY

Overweight and obesity are defined as body weight or body fat above a particular standard often related to height. Three such standards are commonly used.

1. The Expert Committee on Clinical Guidelines for Overweight in Adolescent Preventive Services (Himes and Dietz, 1994) recommends screening by use of body mass index (BMI). BMI is determined by dividing the teen's weight in kilograms by the square of the height in meters (BMI = W/H^2). This measurement correlates well with body fat content in adolescents. A BMI of more than 85 percent for age and gender is considered overweight in the adolescent age group. See the Centers for Disease Control (CDC) website

(www.cdc.gov/growthcharts/) for charts listing BMI by age, weight, height, and sex.

2. In 1998 the National Institutes of Health (NIH) published "Clinical Guidelines for Identification, Evaluation, and Treatment for Overweight and Obesity in Adults."

WEIGHT	BMI RANGE
Underweight	$<18.5 \text{ kg/m}^2$
Normal	$18.5–24.9 \text{ kg/m}^2$
Overweight (pre-obese)	$25–29.9 \text{ kg/m}^2$
Obesity (obese), class 1	$30–34.9 \text{ kg/m}^2$
Obesity (obese), class 2	$35–39.9 \text{ kg/m}^2$
Obesity (obese), class 3	$>40 \text{ kg/m}^2$

How does this information apply to your teen? Let's assume your daughter is five-foot-three and weighs 145 pounds. To most observers, she is a relatively normal-looking teen. She is a little pudgy, and her belly and love handles are visible through her clothes. She is not obese or severely overweight, and common sense would not make us think she is either very overweight or too thin. Now, let's measure her BMI and see where she fits according to scientific definitions.

- To calculate her BMI, begin by converting her weight from pounds into kilograms (1 pound = .453 kilograms) and her height from feet into meters (1 foot = 0.3 meters).
- Multiply 145 pounds by .453 kilograms to get 65.685 kilograms.

- Multiply 5 feet, 3 inches by .3 meters to get 1.59 meters.
- Squaring the height (1.59 meters times 1.59 meters) gives you 2.52.
- Finally, divide the squared height (2.52) into the weight (65.85) to get 26.06.
- With a BMI of 26.06, your daughter is in the overweight, not the obese, range.

This is exactly what we expected from visual observation and description.

3. Body Fat Measurement: This is another scientific technique of determining what we can plainly see. Although real body fat measurement is a laboratory or clinical trial exercise, its use has expanded to nutritionists, doctors' offices, and health clubs. The method uses measurement of the thickness of the skin fold in various areas of the body. The upper arm and waist are commonly used. This scientific formula was developed by Slaughter and colleagues in 1998:

Males: % body fat = 0.735 (triceps + calf) + 1.0
Females: % body fat = 0.610 (triceps + calf) + 5.1

The Teen Weight-Loss Solution has two parts. The first part introduces you and your daughter to a more in-depth level of understanding of how hormones affect her physically and emotionally, and the second part provides the solutions, which involve many important aspects of her life:

diet

exercise

lifestyle

stress management

socialization

supplements

natural progesterone

My plan does not include the use of potentially dangerous drugs, synthetic hormones, or other medications whose long-term effects may be even more damaging to your teen than the problem itself.

Use this book as a guide to help you and your teen navigate through a difficult time without having your stress levels increase or becoming paralyzed by the fear of making mistakes.

By following the solutions in the book, you will help your teen lose weight and understand her body and the changes she is undergoing. Your daughter will become more accepting of the changes that adolescence throws her way, and you will have the tools to offer her the right advice and support in this difficult time of her life.

I must stress that the statistical approaches provide measurements that should only be used as guidelines and placed into the perspective of the reality of the individual being evaluated. BMI is the most reliable of the measurements, but even it does not necessarily address your particular teen's predicament.

It is crucial to look at the teen standing in front of you as an individual and address not only her weight but her whole person.

1

Teen Hormones— The Big Bang

It arrives without warning like a whirlwind bursting into your life and leaving a trail of turmoil. It's a Hormone Storm— Mother Nature's way of announcing the onset of puberty. Your sweet little daughter is now an adolescent. Her physical and emotional presence will never be the same.

Hundreds of hormones are raging through her body—not just insulin, cortisol, and growth hormones, which have been at work inside her from the beginning of life, but now sex hormones— estrogen, progesterone, and testosterone.

Coping with adolescence is a challenge for every parent and teen. A crucial foundation for surviving these difficult years is understanding the role that hormones play in orchestrating the momentous changes taking place within your daughter.

Making the hormone connection is the difference between

surviving well or surrendering to this turmoil and spending the better part of the next decade in teen hell.

The Back Story: When Does the Hormone Story Start?

Life begins with a monumental mix of genetics and hormones. Simplistically stated, an egg and a sperm get together in your womb and forty weeks later become a newborn child.

The master plan, the blueprint for your child, is in the genetic code found in the two cells that start it all. The egg and the sperm come with an astonishingly complex array of instructions for the creation of a human being. There are instructions on how to create and develop every cell of every organ, how to assemble the cells into organs, and how to program the fetus to function outside the womb.

It all translates into this beautiful little girl you hold in amazement in the delivery room, the child you believe is a miracle come true. She certainly is, but to understand her and what she will go through at puberty and adolescence, we must remove some of the mystery.

ASSEMBLY REQUIRED

Creating a child is not unlike assembling a piece of furniture from IKEA. The "how-to" instructions are in the two cells (egg and sperm) we all start from. During the forty weeks in the womb, the instructions are read and the pieces assembled. From the smallest screws—in our case, the cells—to the largest parts (brain, bones, liver, and skin), the body comes together from the blueprint in the sperm and egg. Like the IKEA furniture, it won't be assembled properly unless the instructions are followed. In our case, our hormones supervise and implement the assembly. It takes hundreds of hormones, working together, to transform the miracle into reality.

In the womb, sex hormones determine whether the fetus will be a boy or a girl. As if exhausted by having to make such a momentous decision, the sex hormones then become inert and remain in hibernation until puberty.

This quiescent period is crucial for the healthy development of your child. Sex hormones must stay out of the way to allow the other hormones to get their work done. Organs have to grow, the brain has to mature, and physical strength and fine motor coordination have to develop. Before your bundle of joy can become physically and mentally ready for sex hormones to come into the picture, he or she has to crawl, walk, run, become toilet-trained, stop sucking on a pacifier, and have basic social and verbal skills.

The moment sex hormones wake up and get into the picture everything changes.

This is puberty.

Most often the process of hormonal awakening begins between ages ten and twelve. It can be as early as nine or as late as sixteen, depending on your child. As we describe the process of hormone development in teens later in this chapter, you will see how often this normal variation occurs. Genetic, environmental, dietary, socioeconomic, and innumerable other factors come into play to determine when puberty starts.

WHAT ARE THE PHYSICAL SIGNS THAT HERALD THE AWAKENING OF THE SEX HORMONES?

During a routine pediatric examination, nine-year-old Marcie was found to have a little swelling under her right nipple. Although not usually an alarmist, the pediatrician ordered an ultrasound of the area. Marcie's mother opted to bring her to me.

There was nothing wrong with Marcie. The swelling under her right nipple was normal. Her sex hormones were starting to awaken, and the first visible sign was breast buds. Their appearance on only one side should not have been of serious concern. Sometimes Mother Nature doesn't do things symmetrically. More than 35 percent of the time breast buds appear more prominently on one side.

I often see children entering puberty who have been brought into my office by anxious mothers. Taking their daughters to the pediatrician is often a source of stress rather than reassurance. Many physicians tend to be alarmist, and the profession often over-diagnoses disease instead of offering support and information.

The incidence of breast cancer in ten-year-olds is infinitesimal. A breast infection does not present as a minimally tender lump. It usually is associated with redness, swelling, heat, and pain. When asked, two out of three pediatricians state that they are cautious owing to legal issues rather than patient safety.

Regardless of whether your child is nine or sixteen, the physical signs of sex hormone awakening are similar. They may not appear in the same order in every child, and that does not make her strange, unusual, or sick.

Sex hormone awakening heralds puberty and the teenage years. Following is a list of the most common physical signs that estrogen, progesterone, and testosterone have woken up in your child.

- Appearance of breast buds: Marcie's story is a good example of common reactions to the unexpected appearance of breast buds.
- Appearance of body hair: Armpit hair, pubic hair, hair on the arms and legs, upper lip hair, occasionally facial hair—depending on genetics. The quality of body hair also changes from fuzzy to coarse.

- Change in body shape: Girls start developing hips, breasts, and buttocks. Fat distribution changes. Gone are the cherub cheeks. Replacing them are fuller lips, rounder hips, a more womanly shaped belly, and even love handles.

- Beginning of menstruation: The start of menstruation is the universally recognized defining point of transition from childhood to womanhood. With the beginning of the menstrual cycle, sex hormones have established their permanent stronghold on the female body. The hormones have spoken, and the young woman will now be able to conceive and become physically able to carry on her mission of perpetuating the species.

Gail was a junior in high school and hadn't gotten her period. For a while she told her friends she had a period just to avoid being teased by them. Eventually she asked her mother to take her to a doctor. Gail was a normal sixteen-year-old blond girl. She was five-foot-six and weighed 125 pounds. She had small breasts, pubic and armpit hair, and a very feminine body shape. Her physical appearance was completely normal. The physician she saw examined her and sent her for a battery of blood tests, X-rays, and ultrasounds, looking for something wrong. He could not find anything. He offered to start her on birth control pills to bring on her period or to give her synthetic estrogen shots. Both Gail and her mom refused. Instead, they came to see me.

There was nothing wrong with Gail. Over the years I have seen many girls in Gail's predicament. Her development was totally normal, and the examination and tests supported the obvious physical findings. Genetics and geography have a direct impact on the age at which menstruation begins. The variety of ethnic backgrounds we have in the United States provides a fertile ground for us to observe this situation firsthand. In the chapter on menstruation, I explore these issues further.

I reassured mother and daughter that Gail would get her period when her body was ready and not a moment sooner. I told them both to forget about waiting for the period or ever contemplating measures to bring it on.

I received a call from Gail's mother three months later: Gail had gotten her period without medical help.

WHAT SHOULD BE DONE ABOUT
THE PHYSICAL SIGNS OF PUBERTY?

Nothing. All we must do is acknowledge these signs as normal expressions of the transition from child to adult female and validate the girl who is in the throes of tremendous hormonal changes. Recognizing the enormity of the hormone fluctuations your teen is subjected to can help you understand and become more tolerant of her inexplicable behavior during this time of monumental change.

HOW DO THE PHYSICAL SIGNS
CONNECT TO BEHAVIOR CHANGES?

Hillary was twelve years and three months when she started doing poorly in school. She was in seventh grade when her mother received a frantic call from the school principal. Hillary, who had been a straight-A student, easygoing, and friendly all through elementary school, was suddenly failing three courses. Math had been her favorite subject in sixth grade, and now, only three months into seventh grade, she already had three failing grades in math. Her teachers were disappointed, her parents dumbstruck. When they brought her to see me, Hillary was already in therapy. She had been worked up for ADD, depression, mood disorder, and borderline personality disorder. The two endocrinologists who had consulted on her case concluded that she was insulin-resistant and needed to be treated with Glucophage, which is an insulin-stimulating medication used in the treatment of insulin-resistance in adults. Her parents had no idea what that meant or how it reflected what was going on with their daughter.

Hillary was a sad, plump young teen with streaks of blue running through her beautiful brown curls. She was dressed in torn jeans, and her jewelry consisted of spikes and chains.

Hillary got her period on her twelfth birthday and promptly became a different person. To her parents' great discomfort, she stopped joining the family for dinner, became a heavy-metal fanatic, started seeing a sixteen-year-old boy, and began using foul language.

Successful treatment for Hillary included a combination of changes in her diet and sleep program and supplementation with natural hormones and supplements. It took almost a year to get Hillary back on track. Eventually she returned to being a good student and a polite and caring child, and the diagnosis of insulin-resistance became a bad memory that both Hillary and her parents chose to forget.

Now that you know the physical signs brought on by the hormone changes that herald teenage and adulthood, you probably have already identified the root cause of Hillary's problems. No longer a child, Hillary was led by her hormones into the teen years with a big bang. The world as she knew it, and as her parents and teachers expected it to be, did a 360-degree turn.

What are common behavioral changes that accompany the physical signs that sex hormones have woken up and overtaken your child's life?

- She will not follow your advice.
- She is embarrassed by anything that resembles dependency on you.
- She wants to be her own person even if she has no idea who that is.
- She becomes obsessed with belonging to her school peer group at the exclusion of family.
- She is condescending and adversarial to you and wonderful to her friends.
- She will do anything to make you angry.
- She is reckless.
- She loses interest in school.

IS THERE A WAY TO PREVENT OR FORESTALL WHAT IS ABOUT TO HAPPEN?

Can anything be done to prevent this parental nightmare you now know to be caused by your budding adolescent's hormones?

The answer is a carefully qualified yes. While we certainly cannot prevent the transition from child to adult, nor would we want to, we can moderate its impact, smooth out the edges of the teen years, and certainly protect our teens from becoming overweight, unhappy, and maladjusted adults.

To survive the teen years, both you and your child need education, preparation, and knowledge. Awareness is the start, finding simple solutions that work is the second step, and having a happy, normal teen is the ultimate goal.

Let's continue our exploration of the roles that hormones play in the unfolding picture of adolescence and learn a little more about their effects on your teen.

Insulin and Cortisol: How Their Actions Affect Your Teen

INSULIN

Insulin is as important in your teen's life as it is in the adult's. Produced by a small grapelike gland tucked under the left side of the rib cage called the pancreas, insulin has a key role in sugar (glucose, carbohydrate, carbs, CHO) balance. It is produced and then released from the pancreas into the bloodstream in direct response to rising blood sugar levels.

Whenever we eat, be it a candy bar, a glass of juice, a pretzel, or a full meal, the food is digested through the stomach and intestines and the important nutrients are absorbed into the bloodstream. As a result, sugar levels rise in our bloodstream.

In response to rising sugar levels, insulin is released from the pancreas into the bloodstream. It is insulin's job to push sugar out of the bloodstream and into the cells. We need sugar in our cells to make energy and keep our organs functioning well. If sugar levels become too low, the condition is called hypoglycemia.

When insulin and blood sugar levels work in healthy balance, blood sugar levels are maintained in normal range. When insulin is unable to maintain blood sugar levels in the normal range, we begin to feel ill. If sugar levels are too high, we become woozy and drowsy and our thinking gets fuzzy. Low sugar levels make us shaky and sweaty, our heart starts beating fast, and we're nauseous. If blood sugar levels are either too high or too low, we become sleepy. All people experience low sugar or hypoglycemia when they don't eat on a regular basis.

In time, if the blood sugar level is too high, we become diabetic, and if it's too low, we stay hypoglycemic. Diabetes mismanaged or neglected affects all body organs. Kidneys, eyesight, heart, and nervous and circulatory system problems can lead to neuropathy and even amputation of limbs.

Many people with untreated hypoglycemia may develop diabetes as well over time. That occurs because the body becomes insulin-resistant and sugar levels creep up, owing to years of mismanagement.

If the hormone balance is correct, the right diet is followed, and the system works, then blood sugar levels remain in the normal range, and you feel great. Your body has been fed, your cells have gotten the sugar they need to make fuel, and from the cellular level to the whole-picture level the body is energized and content. Unfortunately, in our culture insulin cannot always perform its function this effectively. Our eating and living habits in 2004 in the United States are far from ideal. We eat processed foods with a great many chemicals, synthetic hormones, and refined sugars.

The foods you eat are as dangerous to your health as smoking! These foods wreak havoc in our bodies and send our insulin spiraling out of control. And all this affects our teens from the very start of their lives.

When your teen grabs a candy bar or takes a swig of Coca-Cola (even sugar-free Coca-Cola), blood sugar levels rise too fast. The more processed and refined the food, the quicker it gets digested and absorbed into the bloodstream and the quicker the blood sugar rises. In response, insulin levels also spike. These spikes in insulin are dangerous. They induce rapid blood sugar level drops and leave us hypoglycemic. We become shaky, have palpitations, get butterflies in our stomachs, get cranky, and even faint or get very sleepy. Besides being very uncomfortable, these symptoms will, over time, produce direct organ damage. Heart disease, brain and circulatory problems, and chronic organ wear and tear develop with continued insulin spikes.

As parents, we are faced with a teen suffering from:

- Exhaustion
- Lack of energy
- Irritability
- Mood swings—depression and anxiety occurring in rapid sequence
- Cloudy thinking
- Sweaty palms
- Butterflies in the stomach
- Palpitations
- Feeling uncomfortable in her own skin

No wonder there is so much concern about the role of insulin and sugar levels. This list of symptoms is only the beginning of what happens if insulin and sugar levels are not evenly balanced throughout the day.

You are now thinking, "This makes so much sense. I knew about insulin and blood sugar for myself, but I never thought it could be affecting my teen. I thought my teen was just being a teen." It *is* your teen being a teen, but unfortunately it is not the healthy way to be a teen.

INSULIN RESISTANCE

In time the constant insult to our blood sugar levels brought on by infrequent and poor eating habits creates a condition called insulin-resistance. Blood sugar levels are no longer affected by insulin. Instead of the rise in insulin in the bloodstream causing the lowering of blood sugar levels, nothing happens. Thus, blood sugar levels are continuously high. Over time this will lead to diabetes.

Georgina was sixteen when I first saw her. She was overweight, short and stocky, and her mother had adult-onset diabetes that did not require insulin. Georgina ate a poor diet consisting of mostly fast foods, and she seldom exercised. Because of Georgina's weight problem and family history, her mother took her to an endocrinologist to make sure she was not yet diabetic. The endocrinologist took bloods and had Georgina undergo a three-hour glucose tolerance test. The diagnosis was insulin-resistance but no diabetes. Both mother and daughter were confused. They did not know what that meant and how it should be treated, if at all. The physician recommended Glucophage, a diabetic medication. Not wanting her daughter to start on medication so early in her life, Georgina's mother came to see me. I immediately advised her on diet and exercise. I agreed with Georgina's mother about the dangers of premature use of medications and embarked on a solid plan to improve Georgina's diet and increase her physical activity. There was a serious caveat to the plan, however: unless it worked fast and didn't affect Georgina's life, she probably would not do it.

Georgina was frightened of diabetes, however, and listened. The results were amazing. Over a period of six months she lost twenty pounds, stopped eating junk, and even started running up five flights of stairs to her apartment three times a day.

Insulin-resistance is common in older people, often with diabetes, whose eating habits have been poor for years. Unfortunately, we see it in our children and teens with increasing frequency. Insulin-resistance develops as a result of eating processed sugars, candy bars, deserts, starches, junk food, and soda. Constantly bombarding our bodies with these foods eventually affects the insulin production by making the pancreas unable to provide either enough insulin or enough high-quality insulin to move the sugars out of the bloodstream into the cells. The result? Diabetic, overweight, unhappy people with high sugar levels who constantly feel sick. The symptoms include shaky, sweaty hands, fatigue, dizziness, confusion, irritability, nausea, vomiting, and even loss of consciousness. The tragedy is that now our teens are becoming the victims of insulin-resistance.

Conventional medicine treats people suffering with the symptoms of insulin-resistance with Glucophage, which theoretically improves the body's ability to respond to insulin. The problem is that Glucophage may be toxic to the liver, an unacceptable side effect.

Insulin-resistance does not have to develop at all. While some people may have a genetic predisposition to diabetes and insulin-resistance, insulin-resistance is mostly an outgrowth of our dismal diet.

The list of woes caused by insulin imbalance should make us all embark on a committed effort to improve our diets immediately rather then waiting to become obese, sick, and unhappy. And it is crucial that we begin with our teens now!

SIMPLE SOLUTIONS TO INSULIN SPIKE PROBLEMS

- Eat regularly—every three hours—three dried pieces of apple or peach or apricot with three almonds or walnuts.

- Drink no soda, neither sugar-free nor regular.
- Increase the protein intake in the diet—fish, chicken, dairy, beans, and nuts are good sources.
- Limit desserts.
- Increase intake of water.
- Limit or dilute fruit juices and power drinks (half water and half juice) beyond one 8-ounce bottle a day.

CORTISOL: THE STRESS HORMONE

Cortisol is a hormone made in the adrenal glands, twin organs that sit on top of the kidneys. The adrenals are part of what is called the endocrine system: the system of organs that produce hormones.

Cortisol is a very potent hormone. Its primary role is to provide protection to maintain the integrity of the body. It defends us from any perceived physical or emotional threat. It is a primitive hormone that has been serving the human body for millions of years, and it functions exactly the same in teens as in adults.

When humans lived in caves and faced physical threats from wild animals and environmental hazards, cortisol was their primary hormonal internal protector. When we're faced with danger, the cortisol released into our bloodstream produces the physiologic responses necessary to help us survive:

- Rapid heart rate
- Increased blood flow to muscles to facilitate running and escape
- Rapid, shallow breathing
- Sweaty palms
- Increased and intense focus on just surviving
- Loss of interest in sex

- Sense of invulnerability
- Loss of appetite
- Repression of allergic reactions
- Decreased inflammatory response
- Change in regularity of menstrual cycle
- Increased ability to run or fight depending on circumstance

Cortisol, also known as the "fight or flight" hormone, is an important participant in the sudden physical and mental changes brought on by stress. Adults already know the devastating effect of stress on their bodies. Too much cortisol released during times of stress directly increases wear and tear on our adrenal, immune, and mental systems. The release of cortisol is important when you're trying to survive an attack or respond to potential physical danger, and it's great when it is appropriately released to get you revved up for a presentation or an important meeting. But it isn't desirable when it makes you shaky and paralyzes you before an important date, a job interview, or before an exam. In the reality of the twenty-first century, balanced and appropriate release of cortisol has become crucial to maintaining good health.

Our bodies need cortisol to stop inflammation and allergic reactions to pollen and other irritants. It also protects us from food and drug allergies by limiting the allergic responses we might otherwise experience when eating strange new foods or taking complex medications. Cortisol in moderate amounts also gives us increased energy and stamina. Ideally, cortisol prevents the body from burning itself out by increasing energy production at the cellular level. However, this is where the positive effects stop.

The human mind has developed far ahead of the human body in our evolution. We live in a world where we receive an enormous amount of physiologic stimulation through the mental input created by the media and our high degree of socialization. Our body reacts to this continuous mental stimulation with the release of cortisol.

The actions of cortisol often fall short of helping and cause more harm than good, especially in teens who are under continuous stress from school, work, family, and friends. Cortisol isn't helpful when it is released to protect your teen from danger that is not life-threatening.

Lucille was fourteen when she became phobic about exams. She was a great student, but with high school approaching, she became tense about her performance. Over a period of weeks she started to vomit before tests and complained of terrible stomach pains. In the mornings she had cramps, lost her appetite, and started losing weight.

Her mother took her to the pediatrician and then to a gastroenterologist. Lucille had numerous X-rays, a gastroscopy, and stomach motility studies. All the tests were negative. The doctors placed Lucille on medications to eliminate the nausea. She became groggy and more anxious about school. Lucille went into therapy. The therapist diagnosed her with severe anxiety disorder and placed her on more medication. Lucille's situation did not improve.

When Lucille's mother brought her to see me, Lucille had a vacant stare and looked drugged. Her face was covered with acne, and she appeared very sad.

It isn't uncommon for teens, in their transition to adulthood, to become victims of severe fluctuations in cortisol levels. These fluctuations are caused by anxiety, fear, embarrassment, and overall stress. Cortisol-induced physical reactions like nausea, headaches, acne, and fatigue are often overlooked in teens as we jump the gun and approach the child with the belief that she is sick.

Lucille's stress level was skyrocketing. Increasing schoolwork, peer pressure, physical changes, and the general fluctuation of hormones typical to teens had added up to a cortisol storm.

A modern-day version of the "fight or flight" mechanism, Lucille's symptoms included nausea, vomiting, bellyaches, and pimples. These were normal reactions to too much cortisol in her system. The thorough medical workup she underwent was negative and did not resolve the problem. Most likely it worsened the problem by adding more stress to the young girl. Treatment with antidepressant medications only clouded the issue further. Their side effects are often more dangerous and long-lasting than their positive effects.

Solutions: Once we knew she did not have any medical problems in urgent need of treatment, my focus was on making Lucille feel better. Lucille and her mother were overwhelmed by the notion that she needed medication and wanted to find a more natural solution.

Once I explained to Lucille and her mother the direct connection between her symptoms and internal fluctuations in hormone balance as a result of stress, they felt more comfortable. Helping them understand that Lucille was not abnormal was also critical. She did not need medications, and she wasn't a freak. She needed to learn how to identify the source of the stress and then learn to deal with it effectively.

Lucille's mother was elated that her daughter was not seriously ill. The mother and daughter agreed to spend time together focused on diminishing Lucille's hormonal reaction to stress. Going over homework and talking to the teachers about ways to support Lucille, helping her improve her confidence, were sure-result first steps in solving the problem. Placing the role of schoolwork into proper perspective also helped. Lucille quickly understood that if she didn't feel well, she could not perform well in school.

A few months later Lucille's life had improved significantly. She was still afraid of exams but no longer vomited before the tests. There was still more that could be done to help her. We needed to work on her diet, sleep, and lifestyle habits.

Apparently Lucille ate infrequently, and mostly fast food and soda. She had classes from 8:00 A.M. till 2:30 P.M. and often skipped lunch. Sleep was not a high priority for her. Both parents worked long hours, and they all had dinner late or on the run.

Lucille learned to evaluate how she felt when she ate better and got more sleep. The results were remarkable. Cutting down on the soda, eating salad at school, and sitting down for a family dinner three times a week helped not only the teen but also her whole family.

Lucille did not need any hormone treatments. Her hormone balance could be improved with stress management tools and the right approach to her diet and lifestyle.

The last time I saw them, Lucille and her mother just came to tell me how happy she was and how well she was doing. She was no longer taking medications, she was able to balance her schoolwork, and her face had cleared up.

LEPTIN

With the rising incidence of obesity in both our adults and teens, leptin is becoming an important hormone. Leptin is produced by fat cells. In young girls the presence of rising leptin levels has been linked to the arrival of menstruation and thus puberty. The more fat cells a girl has, the more leptin is produced. Scientific studies have established leptin's role in weight control, and much research is being conducted around the development of drugs that block leptin production and decrease fat deposition.

Mary and Jane were twelve-year-old twins. Mary was overweight by approximately ten pounds while Jane was very thin. Mary began getting her period at nine while Jane still wasn't menstruating at twelve. Their mother was concerned because she was unsure who was normal. She took them to an endocrinologist, who evaluated them and told their mother they were both normal. The difference was in their leptin levels. Jane had lower levels while Mary's were higher. He made the correct connection between the higher leptin levels and the early puberty in Mary. Jane was also normal but, being thinner, had lower leptin levels and thus had not entered puberty yet. The advice the endocrinologist gave them was to wait and see.

Mary and Jane's mother was my patient and brought the daughters to me. They were both healthy and had no complaints. I echoed the endocrinologist's opinion.

Jane got her period at sixteen. Neither one of the girls developed any medical problems.

There's nothing unusual about the stories in this chapter. While the names are changed, the teens are real, and they bring a crucial foundation to the understanding and survival of the teen years. Hormone changes are the root cause of many of the problems we face when dealing with our teens. Making the hormone connection and addressing it is very important when evaluating the weight problems, menstrual irregularities, and mood swings our teens experience during puberty and adolescence.

2

Natural Hormones

I am always surprised that we fail to see that every age is only part of the continuum of life. All ages are links of the same chain, and they all add up to one life. So why do we separate adults from children and treat the teen years as an aberration? Behavior and physical appearance differ at various ages, but the impact of hormones is constant and continuous. Our hormones have the same names and significance whether we're teenagers or adults. All our hormones interact with one another the same way regardless of how old we are. Hormone action and interaction between hormones is set in stone. What does change is the *quantity* of hormones in our bodies at different ages. And that variation affects their balance.

The Role of Hormones

The proper understanding of the effect and impact of hormones in our teens' physical and emotional development is a key ingredient to being able to help them improve their lives.

- Hormone balance directly affects how we feel physically and mentally, regardless of age.
- Hormones determine the function of body organs in women, men, and teens.
- The individual action of hormones is the same in women, men, and teens.
- If hormones are in balance, teens do not suffer with significant physical problems.
- Genetics, diet, exercise, lifestyle, and environmental factors have a direct and deep impact on hormone function and balance.

Michelle was eleven when she started menstruating and gaining weight. She had been a beautiful, well-proportioned young child, and her mother didn't know how to respond when practically overnight she became a different person. With every passing month, Michelle developed new symptoms. She started to have a mild case of acne, each month she gained another couple of pounds, and her moods became unpredictable.

When I saw the two, I could not help but notice a significant similarity in their physical appearances as well as their personalities. Both mother and daughter were slightly overweight, short and stocky, and had less than perfect complexions. They both had straight black hair and were very friendly.

I saw Michelle on a regular basis for two years. By the time she turned thirteen, there were no surprises for mother and daughter, and they became able to handle the teen years well together. They touch base with me now only on the rare occasions they need my advice.

They learned about reasonable expectations. Genetics was the reason for the weight gain that occurred when Michelle started menstruating. Her mom had experienced the same problem when she started her period. Their diet wasn't ideal—they ate a lot of meat and potatoes and little fruit and vegetables. Once they became aware of the problem, both mother and daughter changed to a healthier diet. The family spent lots of time in front of the TV and very little time moving. They started walking in the local park together every day.

Lastly, both mother and daughter went on natural hormones and supplements and their hormone balance was eventually restored. I placed them on different combinations of hormones and supplements that addressed their individual needs. And they did maintain the good results.

The year 2004 marks my twentieth year in private medical practice. Learning about natural hormones and developing a clinical expertise in them has brought me thousands of patients of all ages. A revelation has been the connection I discovered between mothers and daughters. I noticed with increasing frequency that many adult women go into perimenopause and menopause around the time of their teen daughter's hormonal awakening.

Molly, forty-seven, brought her daughter Elise to see me. She was a tall, fourteen-year-old brunette with pudgy cheeks and a few pimples on her forehead and chin. Molly was concerned about her daughter's weight and was researching physicians when they came to meet with me. She knew I worked with natural hormones and had an integrative approach to medicine, which attracted her. By the time I had finished getting the basic history from Elise and started addressing issues of hormone balance, Molly chimed in and started asking about her own hormone problems. The time spent together turned into a three-way conversation about the similarities and differences between Elise's and Molly's hormone issues.

I prescribed natural hormone therapies for both to help them achieve proper hormone balance. Just as with Michelle and her mother, Elise and Molly needed different combinations of natural hormones and supplements because of their age difference and individual needs. Once the right combinations are provided, the results are remarkably consistent in all age groups.

Estrogen, progesterone, and testosterone work together to help teens and adult women put together the picture we know as female.

Teens are at the beginning of life's journey. Their hormone balance isn't synchronized yet, and they are subject to significant and frequent fluctuations that present often as confusing and sometimes disturbing physical and behavioral changes. Teens and their hormones need to adjust to each other. It takes time to get to the adult configuration of hormone balance that works.

Hormone fluctuations and changes are not exclusive to teenagers. Adult women also undergo hormone fluctuations. For instance, during pregnancy high levels of estrogen and progesterone help the fetus grow and also make the mother glow. The same hormones that make you feel exhausted in the first trimester of the pregnancy, in different quantities, give you enormous energy in the second and third. As we age, our hormone balance changes again, the levels taper off, and their loss is called menopause.

As women enter the perimenopausal years, usually in their forties, hormone changes create symptoms (hot flashes, night sweats, insomnia, loss of libido, weight gain, hair loss, depression, anxiety, and more) that become more severe around age fifty-five when estrogen, progesterone, and testosterone permanently diminish.

The changes that affect mothers and daughters at similar times are no coincidence. While the mother has finished the work of bearing children and raising them to physical independence, the teenage daughter is becoming physically and sexually fit to take over the role of childbearing and perpetuation of our species. The conflicts we see between mothers and daughters at this point are more than just teen-mother squabbles, they are conflicts of survival. Hormones are at the heart of this conflict. One generation is losing them while the other is getting swept away by them.

Natural Hormones and Teens

I have been prescribing natural bioidentical hormones in the form of natural progesterone for teens for many years.

The first time I prescribed natural progesterone, out of desperation, was for my own teenage daughter. After watching her suffer with mood swings, bloating, and severe cramps every month, I started researching the use of natural hormones in young women. At the time I was finding enormous success in older women with estradiol, micronized progesterone, and testosterone for the treatment of hot flashes, night sweats, mood swings, bloating, weight gain, and other symptoms of perimenopause and menopause. Micronized progesterone is a form of natural progesterone made from yam and soy oils. The final product is made out of tiny particles (hence the term "micronized"), a fine powder that contains the active hormone molecules. The seemingly magical resolution of symptoms in adults inspired me to look at their use in teens. Especially when the teen was in my own home.

An extensive body of conventional literature addresses the use of micronized progesterone in pregnant and older women, but not in teens. *Adolescent Health Care: A Practical Guide,* edited by Lawrence S. Neinstein, is a widely used manual in the education of primary care and adolescent medicine physicians in many U.S. medical schools. In the chapter on dysmenorrhea (menstrual cramps) and premenstrual syndrome (PMS), the authors barely touch upon the use of natural progesterone as a therapeutic option. Although they acknowledge estrogen excess and progesterone deficiency as the number-one theory on what causes cramps and PMS, the nine treatment options list natural progesterone at number six. Synthetic birth control pills are option five, and antidepressants are eight and nine.

1. Education
2. Stress management
3. Exercise
4. Vitamin and mineral supplementation
5. Suppression of ovulation (birth control pills)
6. Natural progesterone
7. Medications to suppress symptoms
8. Medications to suppress psychological symptoms
9. Selective serotonin reuptake inhibitors (antidepressants)

Lucy was eighteen when I first saw her. She had been depressed since she entered high school, which coincided with getting her period. She had irregular periods and had been to see her mother's gynecologist at the age of fourteen. He started her on birth control pills to regulate her period, and when the depression worsened, he added Prozac, an antidepressant. Now, four years later, Lucy was not doing well. She had severe acne and migraine headaches and was so depressed that she did not want to go to college. Her mother brought her to me to see if I could put her on natural progesterone and help her.

All I did was take her off the Prozac and the birth control pills.

Within two months Lucy felt well. Gone were the acne, depression, and headaches. She never needed progesterone or any other therapy. Often less is more.

Lucy brings to light a common situation with our teens and the way they are treated in conventional medical settings. When Lucy started menstruating, she had irregular periods. As you may remember from chapter 1, that is not uncommon or abnormal. Periods are often irregular into the early twenties because women do not ovulate each month. It is the presence of ovulation without impregnation that causes periods to be regular. The most important fact in Lucy's history was that she had few symptoms. Her depression could have been managed with natural hormones and omega 3 supplements, as well as dietary changes that included more protein, less fat, and complex carbohydrates. Instead, the gynecologist placed her on birth control pills.

The Use of Birth Control Pills to Regulate Periods

Over the past thirty-five years, birth control pills have become the first-line therapy for regulation of the teen menstrual cycle. Because of the common use of birth control pills, regular periods are now seen as necessary by both teens and their mothers.

If a teen has irregular periods that are not associated with incapacitating symptoms like severe cramps, hemorrhaging, clinical depression, or serious interference with everyday activities, there is no valid medical reason to make the period regular. The only time a woman needs a regular period is to determine the presence of ovulation to see if she can get pregnant.

When we are looking at our teens, their safety and the prevention of problems later in life is of utmost importance. Placing a teen on birth control pills for the sole purpose of regulating her period is a potentially dangerous option. Scientific data on the safety of birth control pills are divided. Although there is some evidence directly connecting the use of birth control pills to infertility, blood clots, and increased incidence of breast cancer, it is the short-term effects that should be immediately disturbing. Weight gain, depression, mood swings, irritability, headaches, migraines, blood clots, acne, and fatigue are frequent complaints that cannot and should not be ignored.

I strongly believe in a wait-and-see attitude. I would rather treat the discomfort of cramps and unpredictable periods with natural progesterone, supplements, and dietary changes than risk the side effects associated with the use of birth control pills.

The patients who follow my advice find that in time, their teens' periods become more regular and they have a sense of security that comes from taking a natural, safer treatment path.

In summary:

- Irregular periods alone do not mean something is wrong with your teen.
- If she has no symptoms, no treatment is needed.

- If the ultrasound and blood results are normal, a wait-and-see approach usually works.
- Treat nuisance-level symptoms like bloating and mood swings with natural progesterone, supplements, diet, and exercise and they often go away after a few days.

One last word on birth control pills. In 2003 a new birth control pill, Seasonale, was brought to the market. It is different from the others because it limits the number of menstruations to two to four times a year. Because Seasonale prevents ovulation, its proponents would have us believe that it serves to preserve eggs for later years, when your teen might want to have children. An additional benefit trumpeted in the Seasonale marketing campaign is that with periods occurring only twice a year, young women don't have to worry about staining their white pants or getting their period on that special vacation.

For physicians like myself whose primary goal is to protect the patient, Seasonale could prove to be dangerous. Going against nature by stopping ovulation and the natural cleansing cycle of menstruation should not be taken lightly.

We are looking at young women with delicate hormone balances. To throw the balance off is to play with fire. My advice to anyone who asks is not to get involved in these types of therapies.

The Natural Hormone Option

Ask people what natural hormones are, and you'll get a variety of answers: "herbal supplements," "hormones that come from animals or plants," "our own hormones", "dietary supplements." Ask where they can be obtained, and the answer is always the same: health food or supplement stores.

Wrong!

Natural hormones are hormones that look molecularly like, and are biologically identical to, the hormones our bodies make. For that reason, they are also known as bioidentical hormones.

Natural hormones are made from soy and yam oils. Although plants are not humans, some of the substances they are made of are similar in structure to human substances. Estradiol and micronized progesterone are perfect example of hormones that can be extracted from plants and are biologically identical to the hormones our bodies make. However, eating the plants or rubbing plant creams on our bodies will not give us the levels of hormones we need to accomplish hormone balance. The plants have to be purified and concentrated to generate the natural hormones the human body can use.

Natural hormones in therapeutic doses (doses strong enough to work) are available only with a doctor's prescription. For teens with mild symptoms, however, natural progesterone in lower doses, available in specific amounts in over-the-counter preparations, are often helpful for short periods of time, when supervised by a knowledgeable clinician.

The term "natural" is misleading because it conjures up images of herbal and alternative therapies. There's nothing "herbal" or "alternative" about natural hormones. They were approved by the U.S. Food and Drug Administration (FDA) and have been available by prescription for almost twenty years.

In spite of their safety and efficacy, natural hormones are not the most commonly used types of hormones. The most frequently prescribed forms of hormones are birth control pills, which contain combinations of synthetic hormones or, rarely, combinations of synthetics and natural hormones.

Unlike natural hormones, synthetic hormones are made from

chemicals. They don't resemble the hormones made by the human body molecularly and biologically. Synthetic hormones are essentially hormone impostors. When introduced into the body, they fool the body into believing it is receiving real hormones. The effect of birth control pills is to override the body's system and prevent ovulation and thus pregnancy.

Problems arise when the body recognizes synthetic hormones as foreign substances and reacts with problematic side effects: headaches, nausea, rashes, mood swings, weight gain, swollen and tender breasts, irregular periods (manifested as spotting or no periods at all), and even more serious problems like blood clots, heart attacks, and cancer.

I first became involved with natural hormones out of personal need and a disappointment with synthetic and herbal alternatives. My purpose was simply to address symptoms of menopause and find safe and effective treatments in an area fraught with controversy and fear. Natural hormones were the solution to my personal problems with hormone imbalance.

Now, after having successfully treated more than five thousand women and teenagers for their symptoms of hormone imbalance, I am convinced of the safety and effectiveness of natural hormones.

Well, if natural hormones are such a panacea, why isn't every doctor prescribing them? The answer is that doctors are not taught about them in medical school or in their postgraduate training. Conventional medicine is still focused on finding illness and then treating it. Natural hormones work best in the area of prevention. They treat symptoms of discomfort in people with no diagnosable illnesses by simply rebalancing their hormones.

Since I started working with natural hormones, much progress has been made. Several books have been published (Christiane

Northrup, *The Wisdom of Menopause;* John Lee, *What Your Doctor May Not Tell You About Premenopause*) that are helping physicians and consumers discover this untapped resource and offering the hope of natural hormones to more people in need.

Are Natural Hormones Safe for Your Teen?

It seems to me, a conventional physician with a burning desire to help teens feel better, that the lack of information and education on the use of natural hormones in teens is an oversight with potentially devastating effects.

Why are we so quick to start every teen on birth control pills for irregular or painful periods, on Prozac at the first sign of depression, or on Glucophage when weight and insulin-resistance become problematic? Why aren't we trying natural hormones that carry a long track record of safety and efficacy? If natural progesterone is good enough to use in pregnant women (a routine treatment for prevention of abortion), why not use it in teens?

Safety issues have not been raised with the use of natural progesterone over long periods of time in any scientific studies. Numerous studies published since the late 1980s report remarkable results, and no studies report dangerous or even mild side effects. Why then aren't we using this benign and effective method routinely?

While the philosophy and politics of health care continue to be debated, I have decided to address the immediate need of the patient, in this case, the teen.

I started with my own daughter. I began by having her use 200 milligrams of micronized progesterone in cream form every evening for the last two weeks of her often erratic cycle. The results astounded me. My morose, snappy, bloated, and short-tempered child lost her edge. Her period wasn't as painful. I repeated the regimen for the next three months. Consistently positive results promptly followed.

Armed with this evidence of remarkable improvement, I started using natural progesterone on selected teens in my practice. The results were nothing short of amazing. And it made sense from the physiologic standpoint.

The problems of bloating, mood swings, PMS, acne, and weight gain are exacerbated right before the teen gets her period because at that time the balance of hormones changes. Progesterone levels drop, and estrogen lags behind and stays at higher levels for a little longer than progesterone. Bathed in estrogen without the balancing effects of progesterone, the body experiences these symptoms. A little natural progesterone introduced into the system goes a long way toward diminishing or even eliminating symptoms.

Charlene was one of the first teens I started on natural progesterone. She was eighteen, and her mother, who was my patient, literally begged me to help her daughter. Charlene was a freshman in college and had irregular periods, headaches, and mood swings. She was also fifteen pounds overweight, and her mom refused to believe the weight had anything to do with college life.

After a thorough blood workup of Charlene's hormone levels, I embarked on a trial of natural progesterone for the last two weeks of Charlene's erratic menstrual cycle. Two weeks later Charlene called from college. She was very happy—she had gotten her period on time. Charlene did so well on the natural progesterone that she started a support group at her college to help guide other girls with similar problems.

Today, almost five years later and with more than five hundred teens under my care, natural progesterone has become an integral part of the program I use to balance hormones and eliminate symptoms in teens. I am sometimes asked, do symptoms disappear because of adding progesterone or because the beginning of the period makes things improve in general?

The answer is a little of both. Getting a period improves things after a couple of days of flow. The cleansing and release brought on by menstruation make many of the symptoms disappear.

However, it is the addition of natural progesterone that helps stabilize the system and balance the hormones so that the period can start and take the symptoms away with it. I also often find that the first two to three days of the period are full of symptoms—headaches, bloating, cramps, nausea. When treated with progesterone for the two weeks before and even into the first two days of the menstruation (for those patients who suffer with symptoms after the period starts), my patients find the symptoms diminished and the periods more tolerable.

What Symptoms in Your Teen Should Be Considered for Treatment with Natural Progesterone?

- Bloating
- Mood swings
- Acne
- Weight gain
- Irregular periods
- Painful periods
- Depression
- Irritability

These symptoms can occur together or alone. There are no contraindications to trying natural progesterone, so even trying it to treat one of the symptoms is reasonable. Before embarking on birth control pills or antidepressants for your teen, ask your physician to try a three-month course of natural progesterone. Side effects are rare but occasionally include heavy periods and fatigue. A more common side effect that should be noted is increased frequency of periods. I often find that girls who haven't had a period in many months, once started on the natural progesterone regimen, start getting periods every couple of weeks. This is not abnormal. The body is setting the hormone balance and may even be "catching up" in the area of hormone balance. The problems disappear with the cessation of the treatment and often diminish once your teen's body gets used to taking them.

How to Approach Your Teen's Doctor About Natural Hormones

Ginger, a seventeen-year-old with irregular periods and mood swings, came to see me with her mother. Ginger was sexually active, and her gynecologist placed her on birth control pills, both to take care of the irregular periods and provide her with contraception. After two cycles on birth control pills, Ginger was in bad shape. She gained ten pounds, her moods were worse than ever, and while her periods were regular, she had also developed incapacitating migraines. The gynecologist recommended another type of birth control pill. Ginger's mother decided to go the natural hormone route because she knew of its gentler approach and lack of side effects. She asked her gynecologist to write a prescription for natural hormones. The doctor was quite open-minded about it but didn't know how to write the prescription.

Since my own patients respond so well to the use of natural progesterone, I now routinely include its use in the treatment protocols that I teach physicians through medical education courses, and patients through lectures and seminars. I am often asked about how the average teen can get access to natural progesterone through her personal physician. Unfortunately, most primary care physicians, pediatricians, and gynecologists are not familiar with the use of natural progesterone. The main reason is lack of available education directed to the physicians. Symptoms common in teens, like PMS, irregular periods, and mood swings, are not often addressed in routine visits to the doctor.

Although the possible hormonal cause for these symptoms is occasionally mentioned in the adolescent medicine textbooks, and treatments with natural progesterone are also sometimes mentioned, birth control pills and antidepressants are still most commonly used in the average medical practice. Only in the more open-minded and integrative practices will you find natural progesterone, vitamins, and supplements being used as a first line of treatment.

My recommendation is to directly raise the question of hormone balance as a potential cause for your teen's problems. Ask your doctor if any of the symptoms your teen is experiencing could be caused by hormone issues. If the doctor agrees with you, ask him/her to write a prescription for a three-month trial with natural progesterone. Do not let your doctor assume you are talking about birth control pills. Advise him/her on the dosages I recommend in the next few pages as a starting point.

There is only one type of commercially available natural progesterone you can get at the pharmacy—the brand name is
Prometrium. It is better than starting with birth control pills. It is
made in peanut oil, so if your teen is allergic to peanuts, you
need compounded progesterone.

Be specific. Ask for micronized progesterone, preferably in
cream form and prescription-strength. Health food stores carry
a few weak progesterone cream preparations. I don't encourage
the use of those products for more than one cycle. Progesterone
is best used under a physician's supervision in prescription-
strength doses. The health food store is for supplements and vitamins. We'll be talking about those in the next chapter.

Starting your teen on natural progesterone is only part of the
answer. Successfully surviving her teen years is a committed effort that involves diet, exercise, lifestyle, supplements, and stress
management.

What Regimen of Natural Hormones Is Right for What Symptoms?

Jennie's mother was on natural hormones for the treatment of
her own menopausal symptoms. She felt great and believed in
their importance in any health maintenance program for
women. When Jennie started experiencing symptoms of hormone imbalance at fifteen, her mother knew exactly what to do.
She turned to natural progesterone. She didn't want to bother
with prescriptions and went to the local health food store and
purchased a tube of natural progesterone for her daughter. The
results were less than Jennie expected. The bloating before her
periods did decrease, but the periods became irregular and her
moods did not improve. At this point Jennie's mom brought

her to see me. The prescription I wrote for natural progesterone in cream form, to be used only in cycles before Jennie's period, worked. The outcome reinforced the need for medically super-vised, prescription-dose use of natural progesterone in teens as well as adult women.

To make it easier for your doctor to prescribe the appropriate doses of natural progesterone, you can show your doctor the doses and preparations I find work best for my patients.

- Start with 200 milligrams of micronized progesterone in transdermal cream form applied to the mid breast bone (where a locket would rest) or inner wrists. Use the same area because absorption is better when you stay with one place.
- Apply every night starting with day fifteen of the cycle (day one is when the period starts).
- Stop using the progesterone the second day of men-strual flow.

Other options for micronized progesterone preparations in-clude:

- Prometrium in 100-milligram or 200-milligram capsule form in peanut oil. Available by prescription from your doctor and available at any pharmacy
- Sublingual tablets-troches
- Sublingual sprays
- Capsules with progesterone powder in them

All of these are available through your physician by prescrip-tion. With the exception of Prometrium, which can be obtained at any pharmacy, the other preparations are available mostly through compounding pharmacies.

Compounding pharmacies are licensed pharmacies where the pharmacist mixes medications to the doctor's specifications on a per prescription basis. There are hundreds of compounding pharmacies around the country. Many of them are part of services offered by regular pharmacies, while others are independent laboratories limited to compounding medications. To locate compounding pharmacies in your area, see the resource section at the end of the book.

Unfortunately, the quality of the final product varies, owing to lack of regulatory supervision. Standardization and consistency of product are key factors to consider when having your prescription filled through a compounding pharmacy.

- Find out how many prescriptions are filled to the same formulations every week. (Fewer than one hundred is not enough to produce standardized products.)
- Ask about the protocols and quality assurance criteria the pharmacy follows.
- Ask who supervises the product manufacturing process and how it is documented. (Make sure it's a licensed pharmacist.)

Regardless of what medication or supplement you decide to give your teen, be sure you are not allowing your insurance company to force you into the cheapest form of product. You want and should only accept the best.

Finally, start your teen on natural progesterone for three cycles. While also addressing the diet, exercise, lifestyle, stress, sleep, and supplements issues, observe the change in her behavior and look at her. Ask her how she feels during the two weeks a month she is taking the progesterone. The results will amaze you, and you will understand the importance of achieving hormone balance in your teen's improvement.

3

Supplements for Teens

Taking supplements is usually associated with growing older and trying to stay young. So why would we even consider giving them to teenagers?

Because their diets are poor and their lifestyles do not lend themselves to healthy living. No matter how hard a parent may try to provide a teen with healthy foods and a regular, disciplined schedule, her hectic life encounters stumbling blocks at every corner. Television, magazines, and the Internet all lure teens to eat junk and be sedentary.

Thirteen years ago I decided to eliminate soda from my house. My children were young, and I believed it to be the right time to rid our diets of junk food. My thirteen-year-old asked me why I had stopped buying soda. I explained that, as a physician and parent, I believed we would all be much healthier without it. Her reaction stuck with me forever. It opened my mind to the thousands of teens I have interacted with over the course of my career. She said: "You don't know what it's like to be a teen today. How can you just make decisions for me?" She was partially right. I didn't know what it was like to live in her body and in her life. I never will. But that doesn't diminish my commitment to helping improve teens' lives then and now. At times that means doing unpopular things. It's a parent's job, and I have never met a successful adult who didn't agree that parental supervision and guidance pay off.

While I cannot go around people's houses and throw the junk food out of their cupboards, I can help teach which foods are good and which supplements help undo the damage done by eating the wrong foods. But remember, even if you are successful at introducing a healthy food regimen at home, chances are that your teenagers will eat junk when they leave the house.

This is why teens need supplements. Their diets are low in the nutrients they need to develop well and to balance their hormones. The irregularity of most teens' eating habits also increases the need for vitamins and supplements.

Janice came to see me at eighteen during her first college break. She was exhausted and had gained seven pounds in two months away from home. Her mother was worried. She wanted me to test Janice for mononucleosis. I ordered a battery of blood tests, mostly to alleviate her mother's worry. As I expected, her test results were totally normal. Away at school for the first time in her life, Janice stayed up all night partying or studying, then sleeping late and not eating anything before 2:00 P.M., and then all she ate was junk food. She drank, smoked pot, and rarely went to the gym. Janice was not unusual. She needed guidance and support to survive the transition from home to school. I started her on supplements, and we spoke at length about how she could best balance her new independent life without getting sick. We came to the conclusion that Janice would come home from school once a month to recharge her batteries and get herself rebalanced.

While many teens cannot afford to go home every month, I find it relatively easy to help them understand how their college lifestyles lead them to weight gain. Once that connection is made, the decision to implement my recommendations is purely personal and a factor of how badly the teen feels.

Choosing Supplements

The category of supplements includes vitamins, enzymes, amino acids, fatty acids, and other elements that naturally participate in chemical reactions in your teen's body and help maintain her body's integrity. As anyone who goes into a health food store knows, there is a dizzying array of choices. Are all supplements worth taking?

The answer is a resounding no. Are any of them worth giving to your teenager? The answer is yes. We will address only the few supplements I consider essential to your teen. Before getting into these essential supplements, I want to explain about supplements a little more.

The terms "supplements" and "supplementation" are part of our everyday vocabulary. Supplementation has become part and parcel of life in the twenty-first century.

The word "supplements" is an abbreviation for "dietary supplementation." Dietary supplementation includes vitamins, minerals, amino acids, enzymes, herbs, and other products derived from animal and plant sources. Supplements are also known as "nutraceuticals." Since it began in the 1960s, the supplement-nutraceutical industry has been growing at staggering rates.

When I refer to supplements in this book, I include vitamins, minerals, amino acids, and enzymes. I rarely work with herbal supplements and as a rule shy away from their use in teens. Herbal supplements have been the mainstay of therapeutics in Asian medicine, but to date their research and use in our Western civilization is far more primitive.

Supplements are not regulated by the Food and Drug Administration because they are considered part of our diets, not medications or drugs. The government does not approve their use in the treatment or cure of any medical condition. This fact is important when making decisions on the use of supplements. I strongly advise you not to use them either personally or for your teen without the supervision and advice of a knowledgeable clinician. The danger with the exclusive use of supplements is that real illnesses could be missed, and treatment with supplements will not cure real medical problems, like hypothyroidism, infections, or significant hormone problems.

Getting Your Teen to Take Supplements

Adults take their supplements first thing in the morning. On the average teenager's schedule, this is not likely to happen.

Jill was thirteen when I first saw her. She was overweight, she was always tired, and her periods were irregular. Her diet consisted of sugar-frosted cereal for breakfast, on those rare occasions when she did have breakfast. Because of school and other social activities, she didn't eat lunch until 3:00 P.M., if at all. She often had a high-protein or regular high-sugar candy bar instead. Dinner was also iffy. Her parents were divorced, and she saw her father once a week. They usually went out to the local diner. Other nights, Jill had either a slice of pizza or a TV dinner while doing her homework. Her diet clearly needed help. Until I could get Jill to incorporate significant changes into her life, I felt it was important to help her start to feel better fast. I had a narrow window of opportunity. Adding a few supplements improved her energy level within a couple of weeks of regular use and made her more receptive to advice.

I started her on three pills every day: L-carnitine (500 milligrams), coenzyme Q_{10} (60 milligrams), and omega-3 (EPA 440 milligrams/DHA 310 milligrams). I have more to say about these supplements later in this chapter.

I told Jill she could take these pills anytime before 4:00 P.M. When I saw her two weeks later, she was smiling. She told me she believed the supplements were giving her energy and she actually took them every day. The results with these supplements are quickly noticed, and the improvement in energy level is often felt within the first week of treatment. We still had to address her eating habits, but now we had opened the door and she had seen results.

The beauty of the supplements I work with in teens is that they do work so quickly. Results are perceptible within a couple of weeks, and that makes the teen, a hard customer to please, more likely to follow my advice.

The occasional doubting Thomas does ask me if the quick improvement might be caused by the placebo effect. I agree that it's always possible that a treatment works because people believe in it. Teens, however, don't particularly believe in any treatment offered by an adult, so that theory doesn't hold. To make sure I am not giving them supplements without reason, I always stop the supplements after a couple of months even if the teen is happy. I watch her for few weeks and then reevaluate her.

If she's feeling good, I don't restart them; if she feels tired again, I do.

I followed Jill for one year. During this time we saw each other every three to six weeks and worked on limiting the processed sugars in her diet, increasing the frequency of her meals, and changing to a high-protein, low-junk, and no-soda diet. By the end of the year she had lost the extra weight, had energy to spare, and was in good spirits.

What Are Reasonable Expectations for Teens?

Mary is committed to keeping her children away from junk food and is a health and exercise fanatic. Every time I see her she tells me about yet another supplement or herb she is trying out. She takes more than twenty vitamins, supplements, and herbal remedies a day. She refuses to go for annual checkups because she doesn't trust physicians. I am an exception because she believes in natural hormones and knows she can only get them through a physician. Mary knows that while I philosophically disagree with her personal approach to health and health care, I will support her because I am committed to and respect her as a person.

Mary brought her daughter Amy to see me.

Amy was a chunky little fourteen-year-old with fiery red curly hair. She was definitely not the athletic type. Mary called before the visit to ask me to help convince Amy that she would lose weight and look better if she took the fifteen or so vitamins Mary recommended for her. I reviewed the proposed list and agreed with Mary that all the items would probably do more good than harm. There are many supplements that theoretically help improve the general nutritional status of the body. However, depending on the individual and the manufacturer, some products get absorbed and used by the body, while others go through the system and come out the other end without providing the user with the desired benefits.

I limit the use of supplements to those products I have researched both through the literature and in my clinical experience, and I only work with manufacturers that meet the highest standards of quality assurance and standardization.

I disagreed with Mary about the likelihood of Amy ever taking all the pills she thought would be necessary to improve her daughter's condition. Amy and I discussed the issue of supplements and addressed her concerns and expectations.

Amy did not feel her weight was a significant problem. She was more interested in having a clear complexion, a fact she hadn't shared with her mother.

We spoke of increasing her water intake and also adding 50 milligrams of vitamin B complex on a daily basis. Amy went home happy, and Mary learned a little more about her daughter.

Reasonable expectations are crucial when trying to persuade your teen to take some of those vitamins and supplements she sees you taking every day. While many adults take twenty pills willingly, teens are less likely to take even one-a-day multivitamin on a regular basis. For this reason, listening to your teen and paying attention to what really concerns her is more important than the overarching need to improve her life.

How Do You Get Your Teen to Take Supplements?

The best way to address supplementation in teens is to keep it to a minimum and use safe and well-researched supplements and vitamins that lead to such remarkable and rapid improvement that the teen will want to take them.

Lindsay's mother read my book *Natural Energy,* which provides a simple solution to the complaint of fatigue so prevalent in our society. The solution includes the Energy Pack, which consists of L-carnitine, an amino acid, and coenzyme Q_{10}, an enzyme integral to energy production at the cellular level. Two years of clinical and scientific literature research helped me develop the plan, which I still recommend and find highly successful.

Lindsay was sixteen. She had suffered with Lyme disease the whole summer and was left with a terrible case of chronic fatigue.

She was one of those rare teens who eats well, keeps a regular schedule, sleeps ten hours every night, and never touches alcohol or cigarettes. She drank ten glasses of water a day and went to the gym every other day. She reminded me more of a forty-five-year-old than a sixteen-year-old. Nevertheless, she refused multivitamins or any other herbal or homeopathic remedies her mother's naturopathic physician offered.

For some reason, she chose to listen to me. I asked her only to take coenzyme Q_{10} and L-carnitine (500 milligrams) for two weeks.

With the almost instant results, Lindsay asked for other supplement recommendations. Our final number was a packet of four pills she took every morning. She felt great and stayed on them for six months. She stopped because she felt fine and got bored taking them. I was in full agreement with her. She now knows that when she gets run down she can start taking the supplements on her own. She knows what to expect and how long to take them for. She is aware of her needs and how supplements work in her body.

The ingredients of the Energy Pack (I provide a physiologic description later in the chapter) can be found at any health food store. I would caution you about the quality of the products you buy. Make sure you get products manufactured by reputable laboratories (see my recommendations at the end of the book).

Solutions: To get your teen to take supplements, she needs to be experiencing the following:

- Feeling ill enough to accept adult help
- Not feeling overwhelmed by the numbers of supplements recommended
- Not being expected to follow a rigid schedule
- Experiencing significant, rapid, and remarkable improvement in symptoms

Don't expect her to take the supplements for a prolonged period of time. She may not need to take supplements and vitamins as often or as consistently as an adult. The goal of supplementation in teens is not to forestall aging but rather to help boost their bodies during times of stress or poor nutrition.

It's not only very helpful to place teens on supplements for limited periods of time, but they tend to like the idea, and I find it to be an easier plan to implement than going into a full-scale diet and life-change program.

I also like to give teens weekends off so that they don't feel pressured to remember to take those darn supplements every day.

I encourage both the teen and the parent to evaluate the results every week and, if they feel the program works, to stay on them. If it's not working, they can reconsider the whole idea, or the individual ingredients, with my help or the help of a knowl-edgeable practitioner.

Finally, I advise parents to take notes, writing down how the teen is doing, what positive or negative changes they see, and how these changes correlate with the new regimen of supplements the teen is taking. Rigidity doesn't work. Commitment, interest, and persistence do.

Which Vitamins and Supplements Does Your Teen Need?

The recommended dietary allowances (RDA) have been considered a benchmark for nutritional adequacy in the United States for the past twenty years. In conjunction with the Food and Nutrition Board of the National Academy of Sciences, the U.S. Department of Agriculture has routinely published a compilation of dietary requirements for adolescents in diet, nutrition, and adolescent medicine manuals.

With the expansion of scientific knowledge regarding the role of nutrients in healthy individuals, the Department of Agriculture developed the dietary reference intakes (DRIs), in the late 1990s. The DRIs include seven nutrient groups:

1. Calcium, vitamin D, phosphorus, magnesium, and fluoride
2. Folate and B vitamins
3. Antioxidants (e.g., vitamin C, vitamin E, selenium, coenzyme Q_{10})
4. Macronutrients (e.g., proteins, fats, carbohydrates)
5. Trace elements (e.g., iron, zinc, iodine)
6. Electrolytes and water
7. Other food components (e.g., fiber, phytoestrogens)

DRIs include several types of reference values to be used when evaluating the nutritional content of foods and supplements. I believe it is important to understand the science and the governmental recommendations behind the use of supplements so that you can make informed decisions for your teens and not become victims of marketing scams that offer no nutritional value or symptom improvement.

To help maintain your teen's hormone balance, improve her metabolism, and clean up toxins in her body in efficient and effective ways, I have compiled a group of supplements and vitamins that effectively and safely accomplish this goal without creating too many complications in your teen's life.

I call them Dr. Erika's Essential Elements for Teens. They contain the following supplements:

- Coenzyme Q_{10} (60 milligrams)
- L-carnitine (500 milligrams)
- B-complex (50 milligrams)
- Omega-3 (EPA 440 milligrams/DHA 310 milligrams)
- Vitamin C (500 milligrams)
- Iron (30 milligrams)
- Magnesium (400 milligrams)
- Calcium citrate/maleate (250 milligrams)

When to Take Supplements: Empty or Full Stomach?

You will note that I recommend some of the supplements be taken on an empty stomach and others on a full stomach. Research shows that absorption rates depend on the state of the stomach: empty or full. Logically we know that absorption on an empty stomach is more rapid, but we must take into consideration how irritating the supplement might be to the stomach if no food is taken along with it. While not all supplements cause stomach irritation, it is important to know which do and to work out a method of administration that is user-friendly and doesn't deter the teen from taking a potentially beneficial supplement. Sometimes the compromise is to take a supplement with food and accept a lower absorption rate while increasing the dose, while other times taking it without food provides good absorption and no stomach irritation.

Here I give you recommendations for doses that work best if taken as advised.

Always pay attention to how you feel, and encourage your teen to do the same. Awareness is key with supplements because their effects (either positive or negative) may not be immediately noticeable and cannot be monitored through conventional testing.

The Essential Elements for Your Teen

VITAMIN C

Vitamin C was the first vitamin to become part of the armamentarium of conventional medicine. Dr. Linus Pauling received a Nobel Prize for his work with this remarkable vitamin. Vitamin C is a premier antioxidant. Its job is to clean up the toxic wastes created by the energy production going on in every cell in your teen's body. As a result, vitamin C is involved in practically every chemical reaction in every cell in the human body. It is involved in the manufacture of blood cells, in the maintenance and improvement of immune function, in the preservation of cellular integrity, and in hormone manufacture and balance. All these functions of vitamin C add up to great protection from disease for your teen. Vitamin C is found naturally in citrus fruit and green vegetables.

Dose Recommendation: 500 milligrams a day in the morning, on an empty stomach.

VITAMIN B COMPLEX

Conventional adolescent medicine manuals recommend the use of vitamin B complex supplementation for all teens. Vitamin B complex contains a combination of vitamins B_1 (thiamine), B_5 (pantothenic acid), B_6 (pyridoxine), B_{12} (cyanocobalamin), and folate. B vitamins are found naturally in animal proteins and animal products such as milk, cheese, and eggs.

Dose Recommendation: 50 milligrams a day in the morning, preferably after breakfast (on a full stomach).

VITAMIN B_1: THIAMINE

Thiamine is a vitamin necessary to help break down proteins, carbohydrates, and fats. It is involved in the energy production cycle at the cellular level. Thiamine is routinely included in food products such as cereals and breads because the processed foods we are accustomed to eating often lack this very important vitamin. It improves intellectual performance and enhances hormone production.

Dose Recommendation: 25 milligrams in the morning after breakfast (on a full stomach) or as part of the B complex.

VITAMIN B_5: PANTOTHENIC ACID

Too much processed food and the use of antibiotics rob our teens of this important vitamin. Routine antibiotic usage to treat acne has increased the incidence of vitamin B_5 deficiency in teens. The symptoms are fatigue, depression, sleep disturbances, frequent infections, and weakness. Vitamin B_5 has an important role in the process of hormone synthesis, and for that reason it is used to treat PMS and stress reactions.

Dose Recommendation: 125 milligrams after breakfast (on a full stomach) or as part of the B complex.

VITAMIN B_6: PYRIDOXINE

This vitamin B is also important in the process of hormone production. Specifically, the type of hormones it is intimately involved with are the "feel good" hormones found in the brain called neurotransmitters. Deficiency is more common than one would expect. It presents with skin problems, rashes, anemia, irritation of the tongue, and cracks around the mouth. Researchers in Japan have discovered that vitamin B_6 deficiency interferes with absorption of omega-3 fatty acids by the body. This is important because omega-3 fatty acids are essential to hormone production and mood balance. Supplementation is used to treat PMS, acne, bloating, and mood disorders in teens.

Dose Recommendation: 51.5 milligrams after breakfast (on a full stomach) or as part of the B complex.

VITAMIN B_{12}: METHYLCOBALAMIN

Also important in the manufacture of hormones and balance, this vitamin is often used to help with sleep disorders and to stimulate immune function.

Dose Recommendation: 100 milligrams after breakfast (on a full stomach) or as part of the B complex.

FOLATE

Folate is another B vitamin whose importance to teen health re-volves around hormone manufacture and balance. It is used for the treatment of PMS and mood and immune system support, and folate deficiency leads to anemia and neurologic problems.

Dose Recommendation: Folic acid preparation 400 micrograms a day (on an empty stomach).

OMEGA-3 FATTY ACIDS

Found originally in fish oil, omega-3 fatty acids are important components of teen dietary supplementation. They work di-rectly at the cellular level to improve mental function, balance moods, strengthen nails, and increase hair shine. In adult medi-cine, clinical studies have shown omega-3 fatty acids to be an ef-fective treatment for depression. They are certainly a more natural option to consider before starting your teen on antide-pressant medication.

Dose Recommendation: EPA 440 milligrams/DHA 310 milligrams a day in the morning (on an empty stomach).

L-CARNITINE

L-carnitine is an important amino acid. It works directly in the cells, in the energy-making factories, the mitochondria. L-carnitine brings fatty acids to the mitochondria and helps the cells make energy and hormones. This amino acid has been ex-tensively studied, and much of the information on it can be found in my book *Natural Energy,* which I wrote after getting extraordinary results in my clinical practice with the use of L-carnitine and coenzyme Q_{10}.

Dose Recommendation: 500 milligrams a day in the morning (on an empty stomach).

COENZYME Q_{10}

The second half (first half is L-carnitine) of what I call the Energy Pack, this enzyme is another important ingredient in energy production at the cellular level. Coenzyme Q_{10} is the ultimate antioxidant and is found in every cell in our body. It is an active participant in the process of energy production and it improves immune function, resulting in heightened protection from infections. For our teens, who are constantly bombarded with potential infectious agents, this supplement is a crucial protector.

Dose Recommendation: 60 milligrams a day in the morning (on an empty stomach).

CALCIUM AND VITAMIN D

Adult women know about the importance of calcium in the maintenance of bone mass as they age. Calcium serves another very important function that directly affects teen wellness. Teens with PMS have been found to have low levels of circulating calcium in the middle of the month when estrogen levels rise. A European clinical study of calcium in women with PMS demonstrated that 466 women who received 1,200 milligrams of calcium supplementation a day with severe to moderate symptoms of PMS experienced a 48 percent reduction in symptoms after three months. Vitamin D is used with calcium to enhance its absorption into the cells. Increased bone mineral density was also found in a study of calcium supplementation in teenage girls.

Dose Recommendation: Calcium 500 milligrams a day, vitamin D 200 milligrams a day, in the evening (on an empty stomach).

IRON

Iron is a metal element that is an integral part of the red cell makeup. Young women often have irregular and heavy bleeding with their menses. Iron is lost in large quantities with the loss of blood experienced at menstruation. Low-grade anemia, often not even measurable in blood tests, can cause fatigue, mood swings, and depression. Iron supplementation increases the body's ability to make red blood cells and corrects this easy-to-miss but serious impediment to peak performance by your teen. *Dose Recommendation: 30 milligrams a day anytime during the day (on a full stomach).*

MULTIVITAMINS

The ubiquitous multivitamin—the number-one bestselling supplement in America—may be a quick fix for your teen if taking more than one pill isn't an option. Since multivitamins usually include numerous vitamins, minerals, and other supplements, even if in low doses, they provide a certain degree of support to your teen's diet. They also provide us, the parents, with a certain sense of security theoretically based on science.

While I am not a great proponent of multivitamins, when it comes to teens I believe every little thing helps. Before choosing a multivitamin, carefully check out its ingredients. If it contains a majority of the essential elements I recommend, encourage your teen to take it. It's a start.

There are many other supplements I could easily add to this list. They would certainly help support your teen and make your life easier when you have little or no input into what she eats or how much sleep she gets.

The teens I care for usually go on a multivitamin and the Dr. Erika's Essential Elements for Teens, which is a packet of a few tablets that contain all the supplements I recommend to teens. The combinations work, and the stress of taking them is limited by having them all in one package.

To summarize, the need for supplements in teens has increased as their diets and lifestyles have worsened. Supplements include vitamins, amino acids, fatty acids, enzymes, and minerals. They do not include medications used to treat specific medical problems.

Sedentary, overweight teens need all the help we can give them to forestall the increasing health risks that their diets and lifestyles are exposing them to.

Safe and reasonable supplementation under careful and caring expert supervision is part and parcel of a preventive health plan.

If you are planning on starting your teen on a regimen of supplements, and your teen is willing to listen to you, I recommend the following combination:

- In the morning on an empty stomach:

  - Coenzyme Q_{10}: 60 milligrams
  - L-carnitine: 500 milligrams
  - Omega-3: DHA 440 milligrams/EPA 310 milligrams
  - Folate: 400 micrograms

- In the afternoon after lunch or a snack:

  - Vitamin B complex: 50 milligrams (includes all the B vitamins)
  - Iron: 30 milligrams

- In the evening before going to bed:

  - Calcium: 500 milligrams
  - Vitamin D: 400 milligrams
  - Vitamin C: 500 milligrams

For those of you whose teen is not very compliant and might totally reject a three-times-a-day regimen, I recommend the following basics:

- In the morning on an empty stomach:

    - Coenzyme Q_{10}: 60 milligrams
    - L-carnitine: 500 milligrams
    - Omega-3: DHA 440 milligrams/EPA 310 milligrams

If over a period of three to four weeks your teen finds improvement in her energy level, try introducing the second and third supplements I've outlined here.

Encourage your teen to become aware of her reactions to supplements, and either continue taking them if she feels better or discontinue them if she is not sure of the results.

Finally, supplements, like medications, are not something your teen must take every day for the rest of her life, so be flexible and teach her to be flexible as well.

4

The Role of
the Menstrual Cycle
in Teen Behavior

The beginning of menstruation is a physical and cultural landmark in the transition from child to woman. The time when a girl starts getting her period has been a source of fascination, fear, and misunderstanding through the centuries. The confusion, uproar, and superstition that menstruation causes to the pubertal girl, members of her family, her friends, and in her social environment is of monumental significance.

I would like to help dispel the mystery surrounding menstruation and offer you the tools of understanding and knowledge so that it does not become a focus of fear for either you or your teen.

To help us understand menstruation, I start with the scientific information we have on the topic. Much of the information that follows is taken from Lawrence Neinstein's *Adolescent Health Care: A Practical Guide,* one of the manuals currently in use in medical schools.

Don't skip over this section. I have made it user-friendly because I believe it will give you great insights into your teen's physical and emotional development and prove very helpful in your
dealings with the medical profession.

The Physiology of Menstruation

The exact trigger of puberty is unknown. The scientific *hypothesis*
for the mechanisms behind it include the following:

1. A progressive decrease in sensitivity to the sex hormones
   by the master gland, the hypothalamus (located in the
   brain)
2. A critical body composition or percentage of body fat
3. An increase in the secretion of specific pituitary
   (second master gland, also in the brain) hormones that
   stimulate sex hormone production

Some statistics are in order because they will make it easier to
grasp the bigger picture of what is happening with our girls. I
recommend that you use statistics cautiously. The information
they give you might apply to populations at large but not necessarily to your particular child.

Onset of menstruation has been reported to occur at about
17 percent body fat, and 22 percent is needed to keep menstruating. In the United States the average age for girls to start menstruating is 12.7 years, with a range of 11 to 15 years.

Menstruation usually starts about 3.3 years after the start of
the pubertal growth spurt. A large cross-sectional, observational
study of more than 17,000 girls conducted by Herman-Giddens
and colleagues in 1997 suggested that puberty is beginning at an

earlier age than previously reported. The hypotheses put forth by both anthropologists and social scientists for this decline in age include:

- Dietary changes—more fatty foods, processed foods, and foods treated with hormones
- Environmental changes—pollutants in the air and in foods
- Genetic mutations—changes in the genetic makeup of humans occurring over time
- Sociological and cultural changes—exposure to overt sexuality in society more than in previous generations directly affecting hormone production and physiologic changes in humans

The study reported that among eight- to nine-year-olds, 7.7 percent of Caucasians and 34.3 percent of African American girls had significant pubic hair growth, and 5 percent of Caucasian girls and 15.4 percent of African American girls had noticeable breast development.

Once menstruation starts, it increases in regularity over the ensuing five to seven years as the cycles change to reach what is called the fertile pattern: the cycles that produce an egg.

The highest incidence of cycles where an egg isn't released (known as anovulatory cycles—significant for the fact that a woman cannot get pregnant during one of these cycles) occur *before* the age of twenty and *after* the age of forty.

Puberty is the period during which the body changes I described in chapter 1 occur under the influence of increasing levels of sex hormones. Puberty is not synonymous with menstruation. A girl can be in puberty and not have started to menstruate yet.

Theoretically she can also get pregnant without having menstruated. If she had sex the first time she ovulated, she could become pregnant. There are reported cases of nine-year-olds getting pregnant this way.

Edna brought Shawna, her thirteen-year-old daughter, to see me because of an unusual problem. Shawna was in eighth grade and was trying to join the varsity basketball team. She was a star athlete, and the coaches wanted her to play varsity. There was one catch.

Admission to the varsity level required fulfillment of certain physical maturity developmental criteria. These criteria follow a statistically based scale of maturity and sexual development called the Tanner Scale. Developed by Dr. James Tanner, it consists of criteria rated from 1 to 5, starting with no sexual development and finishing with adult-level sexual development.

Tanner 1: No sexual characteristics apparent (prepuberty)

Tanner 2: Some armpit hair; light pubic hair; slight nipple enlargement and beginning breast buds

Tanner 3: Increased amount of armpit hair; curly and darker pubic hair; more breast and nipple development

Tanner 4: Increased armpit hair; curlier and more widespread pubic hair; more breast development; nipple appears separate from the rest of breast

Tanner 5: Adult body hair distribution; adult breast development; adult-size sexual organs

The presence of menstruation is a separate criterion that helps raise the applicant's score and helps even if physical maturity is otherwise less than needed to qualify.

Unless a girl is a Tanner 4, most schools will not allow her to participate in varsity-level sports. The logic behind this requirement is to protect smaller girls from physical danger or unusual physical strain. Sometimes, though, the physician must address the individual and go beyond statistical guidelines.

Shawna was a Tanner 3. Although she was African American and was expected to get her period around nine or ten years of age (statistically speaking), she had no period. Her body hair was sparse, and her breast buds were small. Shawna was tall, five-foot-eight, and she had the perfect build for an athlete. She towered over the fourteen- and fifteen-year-olds on the varsity team. Shawna and her mom would have been devastated if I had told them to wait another year. From the risk standpoint, Shawna's physical presence was a risk only to her opponents, so I gave her permission to join the varsity team. She certainly was in puberty, but she was following her own time line for physical maturity development. Many teens do.

By the time Shawna entered high school, she still hadn't begun to menstruate. Her Tanner Scale number had gone up to 4, and still another year passed before she had a period. She was the team's MVP and went to college on a basketball scholarship, where she became all-American. She got her period at sixteen.

What Causes a Girl's Body to Start Menstruating?

Puberty and menstruation are not equivalent. While we don't know why girls go into puberty at any given point, we have more information and insight into the sequence of events that causes menstruation to start.

Significant changes in the interaction between hormone production in the brain, starting with the hypothalamus and the pituitary gland and moving down to the ovaries, must occur in a predetermined sequence to cause menstruation to begin.

The hypothalamus and the pituitary glands are the master glands. Located deep within the brain, the two glands produce hormones that carry messages between them and the sex-hormone-producing glands (ovaries and adrenals). The messages provide information and instructions for the rest of the body organs about the state of their hormone balance and about general body well-being.

At some point in the growth of the teen, both the hypothalamus and pituitary decide it is time to stimulate the ovaries to produce enough estrogen to start the process leading to menstruation. The larger goal of this process is the transformation of the girl into a fertile woman who can reproduce and perpetuate the species.

What Is the Menstrual Cycle?

A menstrual cycle is defined as the period of time from the beginning of one menstrual flow (day one of bleeding, which includes brown staining or spotting that turns to frank blood) to the beginning of the next menstrual flow.

The current scientific understanding of the menstrual cycle breaks it down into three important phases that relate to:

1. The state of the lining of the uterus
2. Hormone production by the ovaries
3. Pituitary hormone release

In the following paragraphs I give you a brief overview of the science behind menstruation. For a more in-depth and still user-friendly description of the hormone interactions, please refer to my book *The Hormone Solution.*

FOLLICULAR PHASE

This is the first half of the cycle, and it lasts between seven and twenty-two days on average. Shorter or longer follicular phases occur and should not be considered abnormal just because they differ from the average. This phase ends when ovulation occurs and the egg is released from the ovary. It is this later phase, the time after ovulation, that determines the length of the menstrual cycle.

Estrogen and progesterone levels are low at the beginning of the follicular phase. Estrogen levels progressively rise, and as a direct result the lining of the uterus increases in thickness.

On the outside, the girl feels great, is in high spirits, and can eat anything without gaining an ounce of weight. This is the best part of the cycle. Estrogen dominates the picture in a good way, and all things feminine thrive.

OVULATION

As a result of major hormone interactions, the egg that has been maturing in the ovary during the follicular phase in an enclosure in the ovary called the follicle is now released into the abdominal cavity. After the egg is released, the follicle, a little bubble containing cells that produce hormones in the ovary, becomes an independently functioning organ called the corpus luteum. Its sole mission is to make progesterone.

At the point in time when the egg is released, the woman becomes fertile because the egg, having been released from the ovary, is ready to be fertilized and travels down the Fallopian tube to land in the uterus, where it waits. The egg waits for only forty-eighty hours. If the sperm finds it and fertilizes it, pregnancy ensues. If the egg doesn't meet the sperm, the egg dies.

In preparation for pregnancy, vaginal secretions increase and the woman's mood starts to change because the hormone balance starts to shift at the time of ovulation. Estrogen is rising, and progesterone follows. The preparatory phase to ovulation brings the hormone balance to a perfect pitch.

If fertilization—the meeting of the egg and sperm—does not take place, the next phase of the menstrual cycle starts.

LUTEAL PHASE

This phase starts after ovulation when fertilization doesn't occur. The luteal phase ends with the beginning of menstrual flow. The length of this phase is pretty much a constant: it lasts fourteen days, plus or minus two days, reflecting the life span of the corpus luteum.

This is the trickiest part of the cycle. Initially all systems are focused on preparing the lining of the uterus for potential implantation of the egg if it is fertilized. If within forty-eight hours of ovulation the egg is not fertilized, the corpus luteum starts to die. The decline lasts until the next period starts. During this time, estrogen and progesterone levels drop, eventually becoming practically nil. When they reach the lowest level, the girl gets her period. During the two weeks of the luteal phase, the estrogen and progesterone levels drop at uneven rates, and this rapid and uneven drop may precipitate significant transformations in the female. When the levels have finally bottomed out and the period has begun, the woman usually starts to feel better.

The behavior we define teens by gets worse during the two weeks of hormone decline right before the period starts.

PMS begins, and bloating, mood swings, irritability, weight gain, fatigue, acne, and even sleep disorders and migraines occur. If these symptoms exist at all during earlier phases of the menstrual cycle, they are very likely to worsen during the luteal phase when the hormones are dropping and their rates of decline are uneven. Symptoms may occur earlier in the cycle because of rapid hormone fluctuations that produce fleeting imbalances. The appearance of symptoms in the first half of the cycle is more common in older women whose hormone balance has become more tenuous and unpredictable.

Finally, it all comes to an end with the beginning of the next menstruation. The hormone levels drop totally out of sight, there is no more estrogen or progesterone to get into balance, and without hormones at all the nice girl returns for at least a week. (It's a little like being a eunuch—no hormones translate into being docile and even-tempered.)

This is the sequence of the hormonal cycle that occurs in a regular ovulatory cycle. Between the start of menstruation and the time when regular ovulatory cycles dominate the picture, a few years pass. These are the adolescent years of confusion when many other teen-related problems occur. During this time cycles are often irregular and anovulatory.

Patient Stories

The following three patient stories reflect the havoc that hormone imbalances often create in the life of our teens. They also exemplify the correlation between symptoms and the cycles we addressed earlier in the chapter. The case studies put a

face and a story to the hard science you have just been subjected to.

LAUREN'S STORY

"I worry about being pregnant every month. Even if I realistically
have no reason to worry, I still do." I had seen Lauren to discuss
her painful periods and weight gain, and these were the words with
which seventeen-year-old Lauren greeted me on our second visit.

Three months before she had gone to the student health center at her college and asked to be placed on birth control pills
because she had irregular periods and terrible cramps. She also
was sexually active, and all her friends were taking the pill. It was
the thing to do. Unfortunately for Lauren, as soon as she started
taking the pill she developed uncomfortable side effects: mood
swings, weight gain, and chronic fatigue.

Lauren was happy she had regular periods, but the weight
gain, mood swings, and exhaustion made her uncomfortable.
The price for gaining peace of mind and being cool by taking the
birth control pills was too high to pay. I advised her to go off the
birth control pills.

After two months off the pill, she had lost ten pounds, but her
periods were painful and irregular again, and the monthly worry
about pregnancy created too much anxiety.

I recommended using a condom to provide her with contraception and protection from sexually transmitted diseases. To
help with her cramps and to balance her hormones, I placed her
on natural progesterone and then added supplements to her
daily routine. In addition, we started talking about her diet, the
frequency of her meals, her self-esteem, and her relationships.

Lauren was in a difficult situation that I frequently see. Her irregular periods and incapacitating cramps were hard to tolerate

when the remedy found in birth control pills was so readily available. Unfortunately, the remedy often comes with terrible side effects and potentially even worse long-term problems. We will discuss birth control pills again later in this chapter.

MINDY'S STORY

Mindy was sixteen and had irregular and uncomfortable periods that had started when she was eleven. Her mother had taken her to an endocrinologist and a gynecologist, and a thorough workup found nothing wrong with her. The solution offered by both physicians was birth control pills to regulate her cycles. Mindy wasn't sexually active and didn't want to go on the pill—she felt fine most of the time anyway.

When I asked her what she thought was the problem, she shrugged. After a few minutes she told me she knew the problem. "I only feel crummy," she said, "when I am about to get a period. For two weeks before it comes, I am bloated, get headaches, can't think straight, and gain ten pounds." Mindy was unusual for the average teen. She made an important connection between time of the month and symptoms and communicated it clearly. Most often when I give lectures in high schools to teens and we talk about these symptoms, girls are not aware of the connection until I make it for them.

Mindy wasn't ill. As we already know from the beginning of this chapter, the long cycles coincided with periods when she didn't ovulate. She felt fine as long as she didn't ovulate. That was because her hormone balance was stable. Estrogen is the feel-good sex hormone, and as long as it is abundant in young women, they feel fine.

Once Mindy ovulated, things changed. The hormone balance started to change. Estrogen and progesterone reached their peak at ovulation, and then once she ovulated and pregnancy did not occur, the hormones started to drop in preparation for the beginning of her period. Unfortunately, the drop was uneven: more estrogen was left in the system while progesterone disappeared more rapidly. During this time, the two-week period before menstruation, she experienced problems.

I treated Mindy with natural progesterone in cream form, 200 milligrams every evening starting as soon as she developed symptoms and ending when her period started. The progesterone was to supplement her diminishing levels of progesterone to help maintain the estrogen-progesterone balance more evenly.

She felt better, and I didn't see her again for years. When I did see her again, she was twenty, her period had become regular, and she wanted to discuss methods of birth control.

JO'S STORY

Jo was thirteen when I first began treating her. She had one period at eleven and had had none since. Her mother had asked her own gynecologist about the significance of this situation and was told that Jo would probably benefit from taking birth control pills to regulate her cycles. Jo didn't complain of any significant problems.

Jo was typical of many girls her age who get infrequent and irregular periods without associated problems. All they have is prolonged follicular phases with no ovulation and without disturbing symptoms like bloating, mood swings, weight gain, depression, or acne. If the teen is okay and has no other issues, I believe in leaving her alone. Her body is adjusting to her internal clock and in time she will start to ovulate and her periods will most likely become more regular.

I didn't place Jo on any medication. We did, however, address her diet by increasing her protein intake and the frequency of her meals, and we focused on introducing regular exercise and stress management into her daily life.

Jo followed up with me two years later. Her periods were still irregular, often coming at six-month intervals. Her mother wanted more definitive guarantees that Jo was healthy.

Although there is no definitive medical literature or research linking irregular periods to long-term infertility or medical problems, both patients and doctors feel obligated to medically investigate girls with irregular periods.

I sent her for a pelvic ultrasound and some baseline hormone blood tests. The results were normal.

Her mother wanted to know how long it would be before we needed to jump-start her periods. "Jump-starting" meant hormones, either natural or synthetic (as in birth control pills).

Much of the need to have regular periods comes from two sources: the desire to alleviate the symptoms of bloating, weight gain, acne, and PMS that are often more than a nuisance to the young girl, and the extolling of the importance of regular periods in the extensive marketing of birth control pills.

The dilemma is always deciding whether to use birth control pills, with their short-term and long-term side effects, or to let nature run its course and use diet, exercise, natural hormones, and supplements to eliminate the symptoms.

My answer is always the same: it all depends on the patient. If the girl feels well and has no significant complaints, then I prefer to just wait.

Sometimes all we need is patience and time. We don't have to *do* anything. The human body is a beautiful mechanism that knows how to balance itself. Just give it the right food, exercise, and tools to handle stress.

What Does It Mean to Have Regular Periods? Does It Matter?

With the new understanding of what happens inside your teen's body once her hormones start to work, we can now address menstruation from a clearer perspective.

- Regular periods usually mean your teen is ovulating, and if she is sexually active, contraception must be a priority.
- If your teen has irregular periods and *no* other symptoms, the irregularity of her periods should not be a source of worry at least until she is twenty years old or she wants to get pregnant. If she is sexually active, she still needs contraception.

Regular periods are not mandatory while your daughter is still a teenager.

Irregular periods are not a sign of illness or a forerunner of problems. The regularity of periods is changing in our teens, and with this change we must adjust our expectations and acquire the knowledge necessary to help them cope and stay healthy.

Studies are under way to evaluate reasons for these changes, and hypotheses for the causes abound.

- Hormone-treated foods may affect human hormone levels and induce irregular periods.
- Environmental pollutants may also be culprits in the changing configuration of our girls' periods.

- Dietary habits that stress our other hormones, like insulin and cortisol (see chapter 1), also affect estrogen and progesterone and thus influence the regularity of periods. I am referring to diets high in processed carbohydrates and fats.
- Life expectancy changes also affect the length of fertility and may be causing changes in menstrual cycles. As women live longer, their fertile years are also longer, and many women choose to delay having children into their late thirties and even forties.

Teen Pregnancy

Adolescent sexual activity has increased significantly and steadily over the past century. Changes in social conditions and cultural mores, and the earlier onset of menstruation have contributed to this situation.

Fifty-one percent of women ages fifteen to nineteen were reported to have had sexual intercourse in 1995. The Centers for Disease Control and Prevention (CDC) reported that 39 percent of ninth-graders had sexual intercourse in 1999. Newer data are being collected, but preliminary numbers show significant increases in the percentages of teens having intercourse at younger ages.

While overall unintended pregnancy rates have been decreasing in the United States, we are still facing an 85 percent unplanned pregnancy rate in adolescents.

Most of the reduction in U.S. teen pregnancy has been attributed to the use of long-term progestin contraceptive methods and delay in the age of start of sexual activity, the latter the result of improved sex education and parent-teen communication.

Contraception

The use of condoms in teens has risen dramatically since the 1980s, owing to increased concern about sexually transmitted diseases (STDs). "The vast majority of adolescents now report using some form of birth control at the time of the first intercourse; 76% of teen-age girls and 72% of teen-age boys used a condom with first coitus," reported Kahn and colleagues in 1999.

Most sexually active U.S. teens today consistently use contraceptives. A survey conducted by the government in 1995 showed that 72 percent of fifteen- to seventeen-year-olds used contraceptives every time they had intercourse. Twenty-three percent of them were using effective methods, and only 4.8 percent never used contraceptives.

The ideal method of contraception for teens must be safe, effective, reversible, inexpensive, convenient, private, and prone to few side effects.

Before we address the issues surrounding birth control pills, we should look at other realities of contraception:

- Every method of contraception is better than unwanted pregnancy.
- There is no ideal contraceptive method.
- The goal is to have options to meet the individual needs of teens, respecting their religious or cultural beliefs and medical conditions.
- Compliance with contraception depends on motivation, education, and understanding. Age-appropriate counseling and education are crucial.
- When placing an adolescent on birth control pills, side effects and noncontraceptive risks and benefits must be

carefully considered by the health care provider and the parent.

Birth Control Pills: Their Use and Abuse

Birth control pills, also known as oral contraceptives (OC), are the most widely used method of reversible contraception in the United States.

The Food and Drug Administration approved the first birth control pill for use in the United States in 1960. This followed years of usage of the pill in Europe, with results that favored use of the pills in the United States.

Starting as early as 1967, reports from the Royal College of General Practitioners in England linked birth control pills to blood clots, strokes, and heart attacks. Studies showing greater health risks to older women who have been on the pill for prolonged periods of time have increased in frequency and consistency of results.

While birth control pills have been refined and contain lower concentrations of synthetic hormones than twenty years ago, they are still made of chemical substances that do not resemble the molecular formula of the body's own sex hormones. They are devised to block the normal body function of ovulation.

Conventional adolescent medicine specialists and gynecologists automatically include the use of birth control pills in the course of treatment of adolescents with irregular periods, severe cramps, acne, or other symptoms of hormone imbalance.

Birth control pills are marketed as safe and effective by their manufacturers and have somehow withstood the test of time. Since no other options have been marketed to the same degree, the public has limited choices. Only women at high risk for complications (smokers and those with a history of blood clots or family history of cancer) are discouraged from taking them.

This situation leaves the parent in a difficult predicament.

Sarah was sixteen and had been taking a combination low-dose birth control pills for two years to treat irregular periods, severe cramps, and heavy bleeding. She had suffered numerous side effects from the pill that necessitated four changes in the type of pill she was taking.

When I saw her, she had so many problems that her mother had made a list for her to bring to me. She had breakthrough bleeding, acne, hair growth on her face and body, increasing weight gain, chronic fatigue, mood swings, depression, swollen, tender breasts, and brown pigmentation on her face and belly.

The adolescent medicine doctor who had placed Sarah on the birth control pills was ready to give up this futile exercise, but Sarah and her mother had read about the safety and convenience of the pill and just wanted to keep trying to find the ideal pill.

I was in total agreement with Sarah's doctor. I believed all the symptoms she was experiencing were direct side effects of the birth control pills. It was clear that Sarah's body was desperately trying to make her notice the damage the pill was inflicting on her.

I practically begged Sarah to stop taking the pill. She agreed, and when we met again two months later all her symptoms had resolved. She was ten pounds lighter, and her eyes had regained their shine.

I treated Sarah with supplements and dietary adjustments and on occasion with natural progesterone (200 milligrams in cream form) before her periods. She has never taken birth control pills again.

I do not like to prescribe birth control pills for the teens and adults I treat for irregular periods, cramps, or any other symptoms of hormone imbalance. I find the frequency of side effects unacceptable.

With every new teen I see who is taking them and is overwhelmed by awful symptoms, I become more convinced that they do more harm than good. Finding alternative methods of contraception is often a difficult issue, but maintaining your teen's health is the most important factor.

Polycystic Ovaries:
Reality, Fear, and Conventional Myths

Polycystic ovary syndrome is a hormonal disorder caused by an imbalance in the pituitary-hypothalamic-ovarian system that is defined by persistent menstrual cycles without ovulation and testosterone excess.

Polycystic ovaries (PCOs) were first diagnosed in the 1930s by two physicians, Irving Stein and Michael Leventhal. Their definition of PCOs included: no periods, excessive hair growth, and obesity associated with ovaries with multiple cysts. The emphasis on the multiple cysts found in the ovaries has diminished in modern times, and now the syndrome includes the following clinical picture:

- High testosterone levels in the blood
- Acne
- Increased facial hair
- No ovulation
- Irregular periods (too few, too many, none)
- Insulin-resistance

- Obesity
- High cholesterol and triglyceride levels

The diagnosis of PCOs is becoming the diagnosis du jour for conventional medicine, even in the absence of many of the criteria. With the increasing incidence of obesity and irregular periods in our teens, this diagnosis is being used more indiscriminately than ever. This situation creates new problems for both teens and their parents.

- Once a diagnosis of PCOs is made, your teen carries the stigma of a disease.
- Conventional medicine treats sick people with medications.
- The treatments for PCOs often include medications with significant side effects: birth control pills to regulate periods, Glucophage (the antidiabetic drug prescribed for insulin-resistance) to increase sensitivity to insulin, and even cholesterol-lowering medications.
- The reason given for instituting such drastic treatments is that people suffering with PCOs are suspected to be at increased risk of heart disease and diabetes.

Mona was diagnosed with PCOs at fourteen. She was obese and had acne, irregular periods, and hair on her face. Her pediatrician sent her for a few blood tests and a glucose tolerance test that reinforced the diagnosis; she was insulin-resistant. Both mother and daughter were devastated. The diagnosis hit them both very hard.

When I saw them, Mona's mother started to cry as she told me of the day the doctor told her daughter she had polycystic ovary syndrome. The doctor told them that Mona was at higher risk of heart disease, diabetes, and stroke. Mona's mother felt totally responsible for her daughter's predicament. The doctor, in Erie, Pennsylvania, started Mona on birth control pills and Glucophage at the time of diagnosis. He said he wanted to make things better immediately.

Unfortunately, things didn't improve, and when Mona and her mom came to see me, Mona had gained another ten pounds, her acne had worsened, and she was depressed.

I stopped all her pills and started Mona on supplements, natural progesterone, and an intensive program of improvement in diet, exercise, and stress management. One year later she had lost thirty pounds, she had no acne, her blood tests were normal, and she didn't carry the diagnosis of PCOs any longer.

We don't really know why we are experiencing a sudden explosion of PCO diagnosis. Scientific speculation includes genetics as a predisposing factor, and treatment is addressed through medications.

Common sense begs to differ. The increase in the diagnosis of PCOs, with its attendant symptoms, appears indelibly connected to our teens' poor dietary habits, to foods filled with hormones, to sedentary living habits, and to increasing stress levels and rapidly rising obesity.

Roberta was sixteen when she was diagnosed with PCOs. She had irregular periods, a weight gain of twenty pounds over two years, acne, high testosterone and cholesterol levels, and some peach fuzz on her face. She had undergone a battery of tests while being shuttled between gynecologist, endocrinologist, and pediatrician. Once the diagnosis was finally made, both Roberta and her mother were partially relieved. They felt the solution would now follow. To their surprise and serious disappointment, the doctors offered little help. Roberta was advised to get into a weight-loss program and come back to see the pediatrician and endocrinologist in three months. The gynecologist offered to start her on birth control pills and Glucophage.

Roberta's mother didn't like the options and brought Roberta to see me. I placed her on natural progesterone (200 milligrams a day in cream form) for two months, while we also worked with her diet, supplement regimen, and lifestyle changes to improve her symptoms. Both mother and daughter felt better because they were being proactive and using natural methods to improve Roberta's condition.

A year later Roberta was doing fine. She had lost ten pounds, her face had cleared, her diet was vastly improved, and her mood was more optimistic. Her periods were still irregular, and she was still carrying the diagnosis of PCOs, but neither mother nor daughter felt lost or without direction or hope.

TREATMENT FOR PCOS

1. Diet: No junk food, no soda, frequent high-protein, complex carbohydrates (vegetables, fruit, cereals) (see chapter 7)
2. Exercise: Increased physical activity on an individually appropriate basis
3. Stress management: Identifying and modifying stressors and individual stress reactions
4. Supplements (see chapter 3)
5. Natural progesterone: 200 to 400 milligrams in cream form every evening in three-week cycles for a minimum of six months

5

Teens, Weight, and Acne

Two of the most important issues in a teenager's life are her weight and the number of pimples on her face.

I would like to believe this statement is an exaggeration, but after twenty years in practice I know it isn't. Teens are obsessed with weight and acne. Their whole personal identity is tied into these two problems.

And they continue to suffer despite all the diet plans and acne remedies on the market. Here's why:

- What works for one person doesn't necessarily work for another.
- We don't understand the root cause of the problem, so we miss the mark on the treatment.

Over the years I have tried numerous diets. I am not overweight, but like most women I always think I can stand to lose five pounds. Because I am in the field of wellness, nutrition has always been of great interest to me. I read every new diet book and very often find myself measuring its effectiveness through personal experimentation. I also evaluate the validity of the diets from a scientific standpoint. I do not follow diets that are faddish or not scientifically sound.

In spite of these precautions, I find the results variable. In my case, high-protein, low-starch, and low-carbohydrate diets work, while low-fat and low-calorie diets do not.

Once on a diet, I follow it religiously for up to three weeks. I stop only if I am not seeing results or I get side effects that overwhelm me (like exhaustion, bloating, fuzzy thinking, or headaches).

I have concluded that if a diet isn't working for me, it is because *my* body isn't responding to it. The same situation holds true with everyone, young and old.

To achieve success with diets, to reach ideal body weight and stay there, we need *body awareness*. Once we've mastered it, ideal body weight maintenance naturally follows.

In this chapter, you will find the tools to help your teen achieve body awareness. Your teen is unique, and once you are able to identify her little quirks, you can share them with her. Once she knows and understands them, she will develop body awareness.

I have developed a simple and user-friendly program for the weight issues. The adult version of the program, found in my book *The 30-Day Natural Hormone Plan,* has worked for over three thousand women. The teen program has worked so far in more than two hundred teens, and because it is integrative and user-friendly, it offers a lifestyle your teen will want to follow because she feels so much better on it.

I believe the root cause of obesity and acne are your teen's hormones. Genetics are part of the hormone imbalance problem. We are born with our genetic code set toward either decent hormone balance or a tendency to imbalance of various degrees. As we grow and environmental factors enter into our lives, the genetically predisposing factors begin to express themselves.

With this in mind, we can help teen girls lose weight and get clear complexions.

Hormones and Weight

Rosalia was fifteen when her parents brought her from Spain to see me in New York. Her mother had read some of my books, and her physician in Spain worked with natural hormones and often consulted with me on difficult patients. Rosalia had olive skin and dark soulful eyes. Her hair fell below her waist in small dark ringlets. She was beautiful. The reason the family brought her to me was that she had gained more than forty pounds in a matter of three short years.

Rosalia weighed two and a half pounds when she was born prematurely. Her childhood was marred by constant problems with colds, flus, ear infections, and tonsillitis. To help boost her immune system, she took many herbal supplements. To keep all bases covered, she also took antibiotics routinely for many years. By the time she was eleven, she had her tonsils and adenoids removed and the infections stopped.

Until the surgery she had been a thin child with poor appetite. Afterward, to her mother's delight, her appetite improved and she started making up for lost time. By age eleven and a half, Rosalia was overweight.

No one in her family had a weight problem, so no one paid attention. They felt it was just baby fat. When her pediatrician told her mother that Rosalia needed to lose some weight, the mother was surprised. She was happy her daughter was finally putting some meat on her bones. So the mother ignored the doctor.

Rosalia got her period before her twelfth birthday. The doctor said that it was a little early and had happened because she was overweight. (Higher body fat content physiologically increases a girl's chances of getting her period earlier.) She was five-foot-three and weighed 125 pounds. The doctor hoped the change in hormones brought on by her period would help her lose the baby fat. It didn't.

By the time she was thirteen, she had gained another twenty pounds. She loved to eat and was such a contented child that her parents hated to say anything about her increasing girth.

Her friends in school were not so kind. While other girls started getting noticed by the boys, Rosalia was just another chubby girl. All her friends were thin and beautiful. Rosalia never complained. Instead she chose to become the class clown.

As the weight problem grew, so did her parents' concern. They took her to an endocrinologist and a specialist in teen obesity. She was given pills, diets, and exercises. Rosalia dutifully tried everything for a few days or even weeks, but then, when nothing happened, was discouraged and gave up.

I worked with Rosalia for six months. I saw her once, and then we worked by phone, e-mail, and fax. She has lost about thirty pounds and tells me she is feeling much better. I find it fascinating that Rosalia tells me that it is only in retrospect that she can tell the difference in how she feels. She is not alone—most patients I care for find that they realize how unwell they felt only when they are feeling better.

In the following pages I will give you the information I gave Rosalia and the outline of the program she followed. Your teen can accomplish the same results without having to travel five thousand miles.

What You Need to Look at Before Deciding on How to Help Your Teen Lose Weight

Before offering therapeutic options to overweight teens, it's important to assess certain critical areas that are often overlooked by both families and the experts helping them.

MOTIVATION

How important is it to your teen to lose weight? Who wants her to lose the weight, you or your daughter?

Remember Amy from chapter 3? She is a perfect example of the importance of motivation: Amy's mother thought she needed to lose weight, but Amy didn't.

Until the teen comes to you and says *she* wants to lose weight, she is not a candidate for any weight-loss program. It cannot and will not work if it is your idea and you are trying to convince her she needs it or embarrassing her into doing it.

FAMILY AND OTHER SOCIAL SUPPORTS

Sofia was eighteen and overweight. She came to see me because she wanted to lose weight. Two of her friends from home had had success with my programs, and she was anxious to start. Sofia was a great candidate from the physical standpoint and in terms of her determination.

She had an enormous handicap, however, that ensured failure. Away at college, she lived in a house with four other girls who were very thin and ate lots of junk and partied into the wee hours every night. Sofia didn't stand a chance.

I wanted to help. Instead of suggesting diet as a primary method of weight loss, I worked on increasing her physical exercise and helping Sofia spend more time away from her house socially. She had lots of other friends on campus, and they weren't all junk-food junkies. I encouraged her to spend more time with the friends who could help her by providing a nutritionally helpful environment for her.

During school vacations the situation was significantly different. Her family was extremely supportive. It was during school breaks that we decided she would focus on her diet.

Sofia did well over a period of two years. It took a long time, but she lost the weight and learned to use her surroundings to help rather than harm her. And the results were permanent. Today, five years later, Sofia has stayed at a healthy weight for her and feels great.

Sofia didn't have problems with her period, and she didn't need hormones to balance her. She used supplements when she was home. In school she told me she often forgot to take her supplements. She believed awareness of her diet and exercise routines and the social aspects of eating were crucial to her success story.

WILLINGNESS TO INCREASE PHYSICAL ACTIVITY

Daphne came from a Greek family. Her mother was a great cook, and cultural traditions involved socializing around the dinner table. The whole family was overweight, but no one seemed to care. Daphne's grandparents lived well into their nineties, and our culture's rigid guidelines for right and wrong eating habits and body size were foreign to her culture.

Daphne's perception of her body changed at sixteen when she started going out with an American boy. When he suggested she needed to lose weight, she was offended at first, but in time she thought that she liked the boy and perhaps he wasn't wrong.

Determined to diet, Daphne approached her mother about it. As you might expect, she didn't get much support. If anything, Mom suggested she lose the boyfriend. Not an option for Daphne.

When I first saw her, I did not feel too optimistic about the prospects of helping her slim down. She did have the motivation, but she lacked family support. Was she willing to start working out? The answer was yes. But change had to be introduced slowly.

Daphne had never been an athlete. She avoided physical education in school like the plague. But her motivation to lose weight won out. Faced with no other logical alternative to weight loss, she started first to walk, then to run, and eventually she was going to the gym three times a week.

Six months later, working out in addition to taking supplements and natural hormones, Daphne had lost fifteen pounds (and to her mother's relief also lost the boyfriend). She now wanted to be an actress and was focusing her energy on rehearsing for her high school play, in which she had a lead role.

Daphne was not only motivated to increase her physical activity but able to find time in her schedule to do so. I often find that some of my teens' very busy school schedules preclude even entertaining the option of going to the gym. For these teens, I recommend increasing physical activities without going to the gym.

Here are some examples of the activities that improve fitness without robbing the teen of time:

- Using stairs and not elevators or escalators
- Walking instead of taking public transportation or rides
- Walking around the house or apartment for ten minutes after every meal before sitting down
- Doing twenty sit-ups every morning
- Sitting up straight, sucking in the stomach, and pushing out the chest
- Bouncing up and down on a chair twenty times, for a minimum of three times a day
- *Moving* as much as possible!

REALISTIC WEIGHT REDUCTION GOALS

Because hormone balances are intimately intertwined with weight problems, many of the teens I see are overweight. But once in a while I get to see a teen who is determined to lose weight with no real reason to do so.

Doreen is a five-feet-tall, 100-pound ball of fire. The seventeen-year-old came to see me to balance her hormones. She had irregular periods, a mild case of acne, and serious mood problems that were worse right before her period.

Starting Doreen on natural hormones was the logical solution, and I didn't spend much time thinking that her low weight might be a sign of other problems. Before she left my office, happy to have gotten the prescription for the natural hormones, Doreen stopped and looking me dead in the eye said: "This stuff you are giving me will help me lose those extra ten pounds I am carrying, right?" I was taken aback by her statement. The last thing Doreen needed was to lose one pound, let alone ten.

Was I dealing with an eating disorder or was Doreen just a case of unreasonable expectations? The answer was somewhere in the middle. Doreen had many family issues to deal with.

Over the following three years Doreen did become almost anorectic for a few months before she went off to college, and she did become an exercise fanatic at other times when she feared her weight was too high. But she survived her teen years in spite of all the problems. In time her body image improved, and feeling better about herself gave her the impetus to develop more reasonable expectations.

The use of natural hormones, combined with supplements, lifestyle change, stress management, and constant support from her family and me, added up to success in a situation that teetered on the edge of failure many times.

Although a hormone prescription does help balance a teen's hormones, we must understand that her life is made up of numerous influences and factors. No one reason can or should be made responsible for a particular outcome. The goal is to provide the best possible combination of hormones, supplements, diets, and lifestyles to tide the teen over while she becomes a healthy adult.

Therapies

DIET

If you ask your pediatrician what to do with your overweight teen, the answer you will usually get is, "Put her on a diet."

Medically supervised and consumer-endorsed diets vary from the extreme, as in the ketogenic diet, to the well-balanced diet that follows the classic food pyramid concept. Here I offer you my input on the most popular diets, with anecdotes exemplifying the typical experiences that my patients and I have had with them.

Ketogenic Diets: Ketogenic diets are extreme diets recommended for very obese teens who have completed their growth.

It is called "ketogenic" because it throws the person who is following it into a starvation state. When the body is starving, it starts breaking down its own muscle, fat, and stored sugars. As a result, by-products of internal tissue breakdown will be found in the bloodstream and the urine. These by-products are called ketones. The higher the ketone value, the more internal breakdown is occurring. The diet is composed of 80 to 100 grams of protein, 25 grams of fat, and 25 grams of carbohydrates a day, for a total of 700 calories a day.

These diets are dangerous and difficult to follow. Often teens who are not seriously obese attempt them, and the results are disappointing if not dangerous. The closest example of this diet is the original Atkins diet. If your teen embarks on this type of diet, even if she stays on it long enough to lose weight, the weight loss will reverse as soon as she returns to her normal eating habits.

Jillian, forty-five, decided that both she and her daughter Margie would go on the original Atkins diet. Margie was seventeen. Jillian's older daughter was getting married in six months' time, and both Jillian and Margie were walking down the aisle. Margie had a BMI of 32 and Jillian's was 38 (qualifying them both as obese).

They chose Atkins because it is the most popular high-protein diet and it works. It also encourages a false sense of freedom by allowing the dieter to eat foods that have been established to be bad for us for years. The dieter can eat bacon, steaks, butter, sour cream—all foods with high fat content.

Although I was not thrilled with the idea, I agreed to stand by in case they needed my help. The first week Margie and Jillian were exhausted, but optimistic—Jillian had lost three pounds, and Margie two. By the fourth week things started to fall apart. Margie partied with her friends and there went the diet—she immediately gained back all the weight she had lost. She was so discouraged that she swore never to go on a diet again. Jillian called me in the middle of the night in the fifth week of the diet with severe pains in her belly. It turned out to be a gallbladder attack.

Margie and Jillian went on the Hormone Balance Diet, spelled out in my book *The 30-Day Natural Hormone Plan.* It's high in protein, low in fat, and high in fiber, including lots of vegetables and fruit. It is the diet segment of a comprehensive program that helps balance hormones in a stepwise fashion through natural hormones, supplementation, diet, exercise, and stress management.

In Margie's case I added natural micronized progesterone, and for Jillian I added estradiol and micronized progesterone, they had different needs owing to their age and circumstances. Three months later they looked so much better. When they came to show me the wedding pictures, they were full of excitement and pride.

Two years after the wedding they have yet to complain about their weight. They are both happy with the lasting effects of their new way of living. While they are both still mildly overweight (using the commonsense approach—they still have love handles and look pleasantly plump), they are not obese and they don't watch their diet. They eat what they have come to know as normal food. They don't follow fad diets, and eating is no longer an obsession for them.

Very Low-Calorie Diets: Very low-calorie diets are diets of 400 to 800 calories a day with supplementation of vitamins and minerals. The only place for these diets is in medical (bariatric) obesity treatment centers. Unfortunately, most people believe they can do it on their own. Especially teens.

Aster, eighteen, was slightly overweight when she read in a

teen magazine that by lowering the number of calories she consumed in a day she could lose up to ten pounds in one week. She had to go to a semiformal dance at her boyfriend's fraternity the following Friday evening, so Monday was the day she started her low-calorie diet. She decided that since she would stay on the diet for only five days, she didn't need to take the supplements or vitamins recommended in the article.

She carefully measured her caloric intake and limited all fluid intake. By the end of the second day she had lost five pounds. All her friends were impressed, and so was Aster. By the fourth day Aster did not go to classes because she was so exhausted she could not get out of bed. When her friends suggested she stop the diet, she stubbornly refused. The next morning Aster's friends found her unresponsive in her bed. They called 911 and took her to the hospital. Ten liters of fluids and large amounts of sugar later, the doctors released Aster after she promised that she would no longer diet. The low-calorie diet, combined with Aster's limited fluid intake, had placed her in a dangerous state of dehydration and hypoglycemia (low blood sugar). So what good was the weight loss in the face of the hospitalization needed to keep her alive?

Glycemic Index Diets: Glycemic index diets rely on the effect that various foods have on blood sugar after their ingestion. All foods are allocated glycemic index values. The lower the glycemic index, the better. Processed foods have high glycemic indices because they get absorbed very rapidly into the bloodstream and raise blood sugar quickly. Natural foods, like vegetables and high-fiber foods, have low glycemic indices because it takes the body a long time to break them down and transform them into the sugar that gets absorbed into the bloodstream. Foods with low glycemic index values keep blood sugar levels steady, and as you may recall from chapter 2, steady blood sugar levels keep the hormone insulin from spiking and carrying with it many other hormones that cause damage to the internal organs. The result of steady insulin and blood sugar levels is a healthy teen, and they also have this side effect: they may even help promote weight loss.

Without focusing on the label "glycemic index" or making lists of the glycemic index of foods, I find myself gravitating anyway toward foods with a low glycemic index. The reason is simple: I always feel better when I eat those foods. Working with my patients, both teens and their mothers, I find that by using foods that are high in fiber and protein—low-glycemic-index foods—I can rapidly and efficiently balance their hormones and weight loss inevitably follows.

Fasting: Taking in fewer than 200 calories a day is defined as fasting. Starvation creates many hormonal and metabolic problems and does not provide satisfactory or consistent weight loss.

New age nutritionists and physicians specializing in extreme diets often recommend detoxification periods during various weight-loss programs. Fasting is often part of the regimen. The 200 calories allowed contain a protein powder with some vitamin and mineral supplementation. The goal, however, is more to detoxify the teen than to encourage lasting weight loss. While I do not often recommend fasts, I do not discourage them as part of a supervised program that is seriously and carefully undertaken under the direction of a caring and knowledgeable expert. The duration of a fast is also critical and should be limited.

Balanced Diets: Balanced diets are those recommended by the American Dietetic Association. Unfortunately, some of the criteria are dated, and the high starch and carbohydrate content they recommend does not allow for significant weight loss.

Judy was fourteen and becoming quite heavy. She could barely fit into a size 14 adult dress, and shopping for clothes was becoming a traumatic experience for both Judy and her mother.

After a tearful conversation over dinner, Judy and her parents decided they needed help with Judy's weight problem. Because they could not afford to go to a nutritionist, the family decided to speak to Judy's school nurse. The nurse was very willing to help and after pulling out the classic food pyramid developed a daily guide for Judy to follow. She also told Judy she needed to increase her physical activity and stop eating junk and soda. Judy and her mother were enthusiastic and left the school nurse's office optimistic.

Three months later I saw Judy. She had gained five pounds on the diet the nurse had prescribed. Both Judy and her mother assured me that they had followed the nurse's advice to a word. No one could understand what happened.

We reviewed the whole program, and I quickly realized that Judy's problem had become exacerbated by her diet. Dutifully following the recommendations in the food pyramid, Judy was eating too many starches. Bread, pasta, potatoes, cereals, and rice were heavily represented at every meal. The result was weight gain, not the desired weight loss.

I limited Judy's starch intake and increased her intake of protein and good carbohydrates (fruits and vegetables), and she started to lose weight within a week. I also found another factor: Judy was dehydrated. The food pyramid does not address the importance of drinking water. Six eight-ounce glasses of water are critical to maintaining hormone balance, clearing out toxins, and, most of all, losing weight.

PHYSICAL ACTIVITY

To accomplish long-lasting weight control in your teen, you must make physical activity an integral part of the program.

- Increase and change the type of your teen's routine physical activity—walking instead of taking transportation, or getting off the bus or train one stop early
- Get involved in an exercise program
- Participate in school athletics

The only question is, how do you get your teen to implement any of these suggestions? It's easier said than done.

Julie was sixteen and spent her early years in Holland. She came to the United States with her parents at the age of twelve. Her weight gain was directly connected to the move to the United States and the sudden increase in junk food in her diet. Before coming here, she had never eaten Kentucky Fried Chicken or Taco Bell tacos. She loved the new foods, and going for a fast-food lunch or after-school snack made her part of the social scene quicker than learning to speak English. Her parents became concerned and brought her to see me after the pediatrician had strongly recommended she stop eating junk food.

I didn't want to throw a wrench into Julie's new life. I also didn't want to just reiterate her pediatrician's prescription but to offer realistic help she would actually use. So I asked Julie if her friends worked out. She nodded vigorously and approvingly. So, thinking I had found the answer, I suggested she join the gym with her friends.

Julie and her mother looked blankly at me. I asked why. They told me that working out was not encouraged in their family—no one ever worked out, and they didn't feel the need to change.

I had to find another way to solve the problem. Would I consider pills? "Many of my friends and their daughters take diet pills," her mother told me innocently.

I found myself in a difficult spot. Eventually I was able to get Julie and her mother to compromise, and together we developed Julie's special program for weight loss. It allowed for junk food once a day, two times a week; increasing physical activity by running up three flights of stairs every day; increasing water intake to six glasses a day (by the way, water was also not part of the Dutch culture Julie was raised with); and adding a few supplements every day.

Julie did well, and I learned a very important lesson. Every teen is unique, and her background is an important piece of the puzzle. A solution has to take into consideration every part of a person's life in order to be effective.

BEHAVIOR MODIFICATION

Any successful weight-loss program must include realistic behavioral modification techniques, but to reach even a limited degree of success, they must be developed according to your individual teen's personality and needs. They include the following:

- *Maintain a journal*—not only about food but about general issues involving well-being.
- *Increase awareness of:*

  - Mood
  - What food and diet represent
  - Family and social mores and their impact on the teen
  - School, peers, TV, and media impact on self-image

- Junk food habits
- Honesty

- *Include food in life but do not make it central to life.*
- *Participate in groups for severely overweight teens.* Groups are often created in hospital and clinic settings to help teens with serious weight problems develop better eating and exercise habits.

CONVENTIONAL MEDICATIONS

There are conventional medical drug options for weight loss that are available by prescription or over the counter. No great studies have been done to show the efficacy or safety of these drugs in teens, or in adults for that matter. Even though many are FDA-approved, the public demand for them is higher than any scientific support for them.

From my professional and personal standpoint, I would like you to know that I do not endorse any of these drugs and do not prescribe them to my patients.

I believe it is important, however, for you to know about them because you may encounter them through physicians, the Internet, or other marketing and advertising venues. For this reason I would like you to be informed.

Most of the following are not approved for use in teens, but with the obesity problem extending to teens, more teens will be exposed to them and many are already taking them.

1. *Anorexigenic drugs:* The use of anorexigenic drugs in adults has been fraught with problems. Serious side effects have forced the removal of d-Fenfluramine (part of Phen-Fen) from the market. Two new drugs,

sibutramine (Meridia) and Orlistat, are being used in adults. Meridia works by theoretically burning fat cells, while Orlistat works by inhibiting fat absorption. They have many serious side effects (uncontrolled bowel release, cramps, and potential liver damage), and the results are not consistent.

2. *Appetite suppressants:* Dexatrim, an over-the-counter decongestant and appetite suppressant, was taken off the market in 2000 owing to reported cases of stroke. Ephedra, an antihistamine, has been linked to strokes and heart problems. Ephedra was an ingredient in Dexatrim and other medications used to treat allergies and cold symptoms. Phentermine (Ionamin) is the only amphetamine-like drug still on the market. It is a prescription medication with serious side effects, including jitteriness, cloudy thinking, and irritability.

3. *Selective serotonin reuptake inhibitors (SSRIs):* SSRIs are the commonly used antidepressants for teens with eating disorders and bingeing tendencies. Their side effects (depression, irritability, mood disorders, menstrual abnormalities, acne, weight gain) are often more serious than the positive effects.

SURGICAL APPROACHES

Bariatric surgery includes four procedures that decrease the stomach's and intestines' capacity for food intake and absorption. Stomach stapling and balloon and rubber banding have the same goal of reducing the capacity of the stomach and thus limiting the amount of food eaten. These procedures are certainly not indicated in teens and should be considered only in life-and-death situations where the young person remains significantly obese and is still gaining weight after years of serious attempts to lose weight by other methods that have failed.

The success in these surgeries is highly dependent on the expertise of the team involved and the commitment of the patient to follow up with vitamin supplementation, exercise, and lifestyle changes.

I will also mention liposuction here. In late 2003 reports of increasing use of liposuction by teens started to surface in the news. This practice is worrisome and irresponsible. No physician should perform liposuction on a teen unless there is a compelling medical reason for the procedure. (I have found no such reason in my experience.) No parent should encourage their teen to undergo liposuction. It is a dangerous procedure, and the fat removed from one area of the body is redeposited in other areas, thus affecting the overall shape of the body. For instance, if liposuction is performed on the bottom, it often comes back on the thighs. If it is removed from the waist, it returns as enlarging love handles and abdominal fat. Liposuction in teens is irresponsible and dangerous.

ALTERNATIVE THERAPIES

Our teens are constantly exposed to advertising from less than reliable sources. They are more susceptible than adults because peer pressure plays a stronger role in their lives. The health food stores, for instance, carry a large array of herbal supplements that promise to help you and your teen lose weight fast. For the most part they don't work and are potentially more harmful than helpful. Since their manufacture is not supervised by any governmental agency, their purity and content are not standardized. Mercenary marketing techniques entice the teen and offer limited if any scientific support to the claims they make.

The typical example of the herbal supplement problem is found in the history of the popular herb ma huang. In the mid-1990s this herb was promoted as the best herbal supplement for weight loss. Every diet pill in health food stores contained this miraculous herb. There was no scientific research to back any of its claims. When users developed serious problems from taking the herb—heart attacks, strokes, stomach problems—it was taken off the market in a hurry.

Unfortunately, this was not soon enough for its victims.

Allowing your teen to embark on a life of constantly searching for a magic solution in the form of a pill or a remedy will ensure failure and frustration.

The best we can do for our teens is to educate them about what causes them to gain weight, making them aware of the connection between habits or foods and weight gain, and then offering them the tools to limit their use of insulting agents.

Commonsense Ways to Protect Your Child and Avoid Using the Medical Profession

I don't want to encourage you to avoid taking your teen to the doctor. I do want you to take responsibility for successfully helping your teen make it through these tough years without unnecessary medications or the need for a medical diagnosis. Before you go to the doctor with your teen because she has gotten heavy and you are at your wit's end, I suggest you take two months and do the following:

- Discuss the weight problem with your teen in a positive way.

- Analyze as many of the potential reasons for her weight problem as you can:

  - Diet—junk food, water, regularity of eating habits
  - Exercise or lack thereof
  - Sleep pattern
  - Stress level and her reaction to it
  - Family relationships and how they affect her
  - Relationships with peers and teachers; school performance
  - Self-image
  - Menstrual regularity

- Commit to working together and supportively improve as many areas of your teen's life as possible before running to the doctor in search of a quick fix.

The solution is in your teen's power, and the help should come from you.

Supplements as Part of Weight Loss

In chapter 3, we addressed the use of supplements in creating a healthy balance in your teen. The use of supplements is not limited to hormone balance and energy production. It is an integral part of the weight loss you are working to help your teen achieve.

The supplements I recommend will help establish a good foundation for the weight-loss program as a whole and should be included from the very start.

- L-carnitine (500 milligrams a day)
- Coenzyme Q_{10} (60 milligrams a day)
- Omega-3 fatty acids (DHA 440 milligrams/EPA 310 milligrams a day)
- Vitamin B complex (50 milligrams a day)
- Calcium (250 milligrams a day)
- Magnesium (400 milligrams a day)
- Zinc (25 milligrams a day)

Start your teen on them on the first day of the balancing weight reduction plan.

Hormones and Weight Gain

When we talk about the balance of hormones and primarily the imbalances associated with teenagers, we invariably look at the enormous problem of weight gain. It is infrequent to find a teen with hormone imbalances who has not experienced weight gain or difficulties losing weight.

As you start your teen on the weight-loss program outlined here, you must keep in mind the hormone connection. *No diet or exercise program will be effective and accomplish the desired weight loss if the teen's hormones are out of balance.*

Before starting the diet, exercise, supplements, and lifestyle changes, take your teen to the doctor and have her hormone balance evaluated. If she is overweight and also has irregular periods, cramps, bloating, headaches, acne, and mood swings, you are looking at a hormone-rooted problem that needs solving before your teen can lose the weight or rid herself of acne.

In chapters 1 and 2, we learned about hormone balance, and I would strongly recommend addressing these problems with your doctor. To ensure success in the weight reduction program, your teen's hormones have to be balanced.

Synthetic birth control pills will not balance hormones.

Diet and exercise with the right supplements will help. Adding natural progesterone (200 milligrams a day) for two weeks a month for three to six months will greatly increase the chances for success. I look at the natural progesterone connection as a crucial link in the chain of good health and balance for your teen.

Hormones and Acne: Is There a Connection?

Clarisse, fourteen, had beautiful clear skin until three months after she started menstruating. She went from perfect skin to a face covered with pimples in a matter of weeks. Her forehead and chin were constantly under siege. Clarisse saw a dermatologist and was given a few types of skin cleansers and topical antibiotics. The improvement was minimal, and after three visits the dermatologist decided Clarisse had *no* choice but to start Accutane. Accutane is a very potent drug. It requires regular blood tests because of its potential side effect of damage to the liver. Accutane is so dangerous to unborn babies that it is never given to sexually active women unless they are on birth control pills and have a negative pregnancy test before the prescription is started.

Clarisse's mother felt uncomfortable and brought Clarisse to see me. I agreed with her. No matter how bad the acne was (and I have certainly seen worse), giving a fourteen-year-old this drug seemed drastic to me. When asked about Clarisse's diet regimen, I found out that she had a sweet tooth and her diet consisted mostly of junk food and soda. She ate only once a day. She skipped lunch, ate dinner, and drank very little water. She did not exercise regularly, and her school stress level was very high.

Clarisse's story is common. Acne is a symptom of hormone imbalance. When girls and boys enter puberty and their sex hormones awaken, their physical body undergoes enormous changes. While the balance of hormones is uneven and unsettled in the early years of puberty, it isn't uncommon to develop acne.

I treated Clarisse with a combination program. The program, individually adapted to fit a particular teen's need, is simple and works. Try it with your teen:

- Increase water intake. (Send her to school with a bottle of water).
- Decrease soda intake. (Whatever amount she drinks now, decrease it by one every other day until she doesn't drink soda anymore. Don't keep it in the house.)
- Limit the amount of junk food. (One visit to McDonald's, Burger King, or Taco Bell a week).
- Increase meal frequency. (Include snacks of dried fruit and almonds and walnuts every three hours. Put them in a plastic bag and throw it into her backpack or have her make her own. Share the good stuff!)
- Increase physical activity. (This doesn't have to be formal gym or athletics. Moving is enough in teens who are sedentary.)
- Help improve her sleep pattern. (As much as possible make the bedroom a space to rest and sleep.)
- Use selected supplements. They do work and help clear up the skin from the inside out (L-carnitine [500 milligrams a day], coenzyme Q_{10} [60 milligrams a day], omega-3 [DHA 440 milligrams/EPA 310 milligrams a

day], vitamin B complex [50 milligrams a day], DMAE [50 milligrams a day]). When she feels better, she will want to continue taking them.

- Give her natural progesterone every evening for the two weeks before her period.
- Acknowledge and decrease the impact that stress has on her body. (Unless you talk to her and point out the obvious connections, she may not see them and you may be missing an important opportunity to help.)
- Help her improve her positive expectations. (Expect things to get better. Be confident that you are helping her and she will do better. Just make sure you actually implement all the above.)

Clarisse's skin cleared within a period of three months and has been free of acne for the past two years.

Weight and acne are serious problems in our teens. In these few pages I have condensed as much information as I could to give you the insight and information you need to help your teen. Resolving the issues of weight and hormone imbalances in adolescents takes time and is an ongoing process. Understanding the process, helping your child develop self-awareness, and offering tools that lead to improvement are part of the formula for success we are all striving for.

6

Teen Identity
and the Hormone
Connection

My area of expertise is medical, and I focus on hormone imbalances—how they affect weight and create uncomfortable symptoms. I often see teens with behavioral problems as well, however, because many teens with hormone imbalances also have issues with social interaction and personal identity.

Jane came to my office in desperation. She was looking for help in managing her seventeen-year-old daughter Roseanne after three years of futile visits to psychologists, nutritionists, endocrinologists, and adolescent medicine specialists.

The last stop had been an integrative medical program that included visits with various specialists three times a week. For her problems with depression and mood swings, Roseanne was taking Prozac, and for her irregular and painful periods, she was on birth control pills. Now, besides feeling awful, she was behaving badly and looked terrible. Jane was at her wit's end. She was a single mother, had two jobs, and offered her two children a comfortable, stable life.

Roseanne had been a model child until she turned fourteen. At that point she started skipping school, hanging out with the wrong crowd, and verbally and emotionally abusing her mother and younger brother.

She stayed up all night and slept all day. Guidance counselors and school psychologists found all kinds of reasons why Roseanne was acting out, but they could not come up with solutions.

Roseanne's parents had divorced when she was three, but her father lived close by and saw her on a regular basis. Jane felt she had a good support system to help raise her children. She was well educated and read many books on child-rearing. At the first sign of trouble she had gone to the school psychologist to ask for help with her daughter. Her commitment was unwavering. No matter how bad things got, she was not going to give up. She just felt lost at this point and didn't know which way to turn.

I felt sad for both of them. They weren't speaking the same language, and they were both in pain. Jane told me that therapy made them both feel inadequate and abnormal. Her daughter was in trouble physically and emotionally, and Jane hadn't found the tools to help. "I can't manage her," she said.

Roseanne's biggest problem with her mother was: "She won't listen to me."

I often see mother-daughter teams in similar situations. Lost in our health-care system and desperately looking for solutions, they find more complications that give rise to increased confusion and fear. My goal is to offer solutions, not criticisms, so I will not linger on the negatives.

Teen Identity

What is really going on and how can we help? Simply stated, your teen is trying to figure out who she is.

When Roseanne was a child, she knew exactly who she was. She had blue eyes, and she liked cookies, steak, and hot dogs. She was going to become a ballerina, a doctor, a mom. She didn't need much input from the outside world to be sure.

Suddenly, when her hormones began to work and her body started to visibly change, the little girl turned into a teen and her identity vanished. When puberty starts and the hormones instigate this transformation of cataclysmic proportions (see chapter 1), the girl's clear image of herself disappears almost overnight.

A great description of the dramatic loss of identity that occurs in the period of transition from child to adolescent can be found in *An American Childhood* by Annie Dillard. Although the book was published more than fifteen years ago, it still gives topical insights into what happens to your little girl who unequivocally knew who she was at ten but has no idea who she is at fourteen. Since Annie Dillard's book was published, there have been a few others that explore the magical disappearance of a girl's identity into the confusion started by the beginning of adolescence and continued for the better part of a woman's adult life. This sudden change is directly connected to the physical changes brought on by the action of hormones.

Is the Influence of Hormones a Life Sentence?

If we look at our lives physiologically from puberty to menopause, the common thread is the constant and continuous influence of our hormones on how we feel, how we look, and how we react to our world. If we can understand that impact, if we can develop the awareness and obtain the tools to harness the hormones and keep them in balance, we can live healthy and satisfying lives. If we miss out on the opportunity to identify and treat symptoms of hormone imbalance and become victims of vicious life cycles we develop in our youth, we are doomed to a life of weight, mood, and myriad other hormone-related problems.

For this reason alone, we must teach our teens from the beginning how to identify potential problems and use safe solutions that will work for a lifetime. Once we understand and incorporate this immutable logic, we can help our adolescents and ourselves at the same time.

Before I give you the tools and outline the solutions, I want to tell you what happened to Jane and Roseanne.

We started by agreeing that both were right.

Jane rightfully believed she needed parental control over her daughter's life. Roseanne was not mature enough to lead an independent life, and when presented with the reality that she needed financial support, an education, and an ability to prioritize and solve problems, she agreed she needed her mom.

Jane also had to agree that she wasn't listening to her daughter's needs because she did not trust her daughter's judgment and was also disappointed in her behavior and performance.

Once we had agreement from both sides on the validity of their individual complaints, we moved ahead quickly.

We looked at Roseanne's life and her expectations. Within a couple of visits it became apparent to both mother and daughter that Roseanne was torn between wanting to still be a little girl and wanting to appear independent and grown-up in front of her peer group.

So we made a pact.

- Roseanne and Jane would spend time together away from anyone else once a week. They would go shopping, go out for a meal, or just sit around and talk.
- Jane would not pass judgment, and Roseanne would not be condescending or offensive to her mother.
- At first they talked about the weather, but in time they started to talk about what was going on in Roseanne's life—boys, girls, drugs, sex, school. Sometimes their talks ended in arguments, but mostly they did not.
- Roseanne and Jane, with my help, addressed their diets and improved them to ensure better hormone balance.
- Mother and daughter became aware of the need to lead more disciplined, organized lives, and together they devised a plan for regular dinners and family time.
- They started taking supplements and natural hormones under my supervision.

One year later, when I last saw Roseanne and Jane, they were both quite satisfied with the results. Although they were not totally solved, their problems had significantly diminished. They were now getting along, Roseanne was doing well in school, and her peer group had changed slightly, but for the better. Roseanne was no longer taking medication or birth control pills, and she had abandoned the three-times-a-week therapy sessions. She still saw her psychologist every few weeks just to check in.

Above all, there was no sense of desperation, and both mother and daughter now understood that they needed time to grow and heal.

Why Do We Have Trouble with Teens?

We expect them to behave like adults and they are not adults.

This sentence summarizes the biggest problem we have with our teens. The second they stop looking like children, we throw adult expectations at them, whether for behavior, intelligence, problem-solving abilities, you name it.

We need to realize that although physically they may look like adults, emotionally they are far from being adults.

The sudden surge of sex hormones in their bodies has created tremendous and rapid changes. Their physical appearance has turned them into sexual, physically mature people, while their emotional and mental development is still somewhere at the tail end of childhood.

The importance of the hormone connection cannot be overemphasized. I can state with certainty that the root cause of the problems we have with our teens is the activation of the hormones, which changes the entire picture. The emotional and behavioral problems that develop occur along with the hormone changes.

To help teens gain better understanding of their identity, we need to change a cultural and educational paradigm. We have to stop separating the mind from the body.

We must accept that our hormones define our teens both physically and psychologically.

How can we help?

The solution involves five steps:

1. Gaining awareness of the source of the problem— sudden hormone changes.

2. Seeing teens realistically—many parents don't want to admit to the truth about their children and would rather see them through rose-colored glasses.

3. Managing expectations—teens are not adults, even though they look like adults, so we can't treat them like adults.

4. Working with teens in an environment that supports and encourages their personal development and growth—they need their parents for guidelines, boundaries, and rules.

5. Making a commitment to success—regardless of how discouraging or painful situations may get, the parent must make the commitment to help the teen successfully negotiate the transition.

Following these guidelines may not solve every single problem with your teenager, but it will certainly increase your chances for success.

After twenty years in private practice, using concrete medical and integrative solutions and better awareness of the connection between body and mind, I find this approach almost foolproof in the treatment of teens.

Isabella was sixteen when her mother brought her to see me. The family came from Italy, and they were very closely knit. Rebellion was not an option in her culture. Children listened to their parents and no one spoke back.

Isabella was being raised between New Bedford, Massachusetts, where she lived with her parents and went to school, and Pessaro, Italy, where she spent her summers with her grandparents. One day in the winter of her sixteenth year, Isabella got on a plane and flew to Italy without telling anyone where she was going. According to her mother, one day she was in school, doing relatively well, and the next day she just disappeared.

Fortunately, her grandmother called with the news of her granddaughter's unexpected arrival just at the time when her parents were starting to panic.

Her mother flew to Italy to bring her back. Initially the parents were relieved that Isabella was physically all right, but once they were safely on the plane, things started to change. Isabella became angry and morose and announced that she would run away again. She hated living with her parents and wanted to go back to Italy. Her mother became furious with Isabella and threatened to turn her over to her father, who was from the old country and wasn't afraid of corporal punishment. Isabella and her mother were at a serious impasse.

Isabella's mother decided her daughter needed help and took her to a pediatrician, who recommended psychiatric counseling and medication. Isabella's mother didn't like that option and came to see me.

During a thorough review of the history, it became clear that Isabella's change in personality started with the beginning of her menstruation. She had been perfectly happy until age fourteen. She was slow to develop, as she told me herself, but that didn't bother her. Once she started growing breasts and getting pubic hair, she began to feel awkward.

When her period started, she became totally confused. She didn't like it at all. The pressure that came with the period was too much for her to handle. She had to worry about boys, how she looked, her weight, her friends; her whole life came crashing down on her.

She was sure she told her mother she was unhappy. Her mother did not remember. The mother believed she was being totally understanding and supportive of her daughter's changing needs. She proudly told me she took Isabella for her first facial, had her hair highlighted, and even spent a week with her at a spa in the Catskills. Not exactly what Isabella wanted.

Isabella didn't want to grow up so fast. She didn't want to disappoint her mother, but she was not ready to be a "sexy teen," as she called her mother's expectations. She still wanted to be a child. For that reason, she went back to Italy, where she felt no one would pressure her to grow up, where she could still be a child.

Once our conversation began to uncover the root cause of Isabella's change, both Isabella and her mother relaxed.

Isabella was not a freak. She was a normal teen who was not yet ready to be an adult. It wasn't Isabella who was at fault; it was the system around her pushing her to be someone she wasn't ready to be. With the best intentions, her mother was reacting to cultural peer pressure instead of to her own daughter's needs.

No one runs away from too much good. Something is wrong when teens start to seriously act out! The key is to figure out why they are acting out before it snowballs and you lose control of the situation.

I believe a key starting point is to take responsibility and acknowledge that things are not okay when they aren't. The head-in-the-sand approach doesn't work.

I worked with Isabella and her mother for almost a year in the following areas:

- I made them both aware that the change in Isabella started with the onset of puberty and the beginning of her period. Once her sex hormones (estrogen and progesterone) woke up and became active, they changed her physical appearance so that she no longer looked like a child but rather started to look like a young woman. This physical change led to a change in the way she was viewed by her peers and family. The result was increased peer pressure and family expectations for her to be acting like a woman. For Isabella, this change in expectations occurred too fast. She wasn't ready. She thought she had tried to communicate her feelings to her mother, but her mother's reaction wasn't what she expected. Being a teen, she had no other tools for coping, and so she ran away to Italy, where she could be a child again.

- We worked with diet, stress management, supplements, and natural hormones to help make the hormone transition easier and less stressful on Isabella's body and mind. The role of the supplements and natural hormones was to balance the emotional and physical changes that caused her so much difficulty. Being educated about diet, stress management, and exercise helped her integrate all segments of her life into the new person she was becoming. Teaching her body an identity awareness was the goal. In time Isabella became accustomed to the new person she had become and came to see the changes not as strange and scary but rather as normal.

- I taught Isabella's mother to see her teen as a unique person, not an extension of herself or the teens she saw in magazines or on TV. Eager to please and support her daughter, Isabella's mother made a mistake I often see in my practice with teens: she neglected to notice Isabella. Instead of addressing Isabella's individual issues and doubts, she took her lead from the media, not her child. While this approach often works, because most teens are very susceptible to peer and celebrity leads, in Isabella's case it wasn't helpful.

- I helped Isabella understand that her mother was totally committed to making things work for her. Isabella was faced with her mother's lack of understanding for her and ran away from her mother's pressure. She didn't realize that her mother had the best intentions at heart. Once Isabella understood that communicating with her mother took work but brought her great support and emotional rewards, she stopped running, and the two started sharing information and support.

It all worked out well for Isabella. She never ran away from home again. She refocused her fear of having to compete in the "sexy girl" category by becoming a star athlete. She joined the school soccer team and became its captain by senior year.

Not every teen girl will become sexually active or a bombshell when she turns into an adolescent, nor should she have to. In spite of the pictures and stories we read in magazines and watch on television, becoming Britney Spears isn't an obligatory transition into adulthood.

It's okay not to want to fit into that mold. Often it is even better.

Support and encouragement from you, the parent, will validate your teen's individuality and allow her to be herself. Realistic and honest support is part and parcel of your commitment to her, and her development of a solid self-image is the reward.

A parent's blind agreement, however, can be detrimental.

Cindy was sixteen when I first saw her. She wanted help regulating her periods. She was taking birth control pills and was sexually active. Her face was covered with pimples, and she was at least fifteen pounds overweight. She wore a lot of makeup and revealing clothing.

Her mother came along for her visit. A slight, mousy-looking woman, Cindy's mom believed herself to be the ideal, supportive mother. She told me she knew all about Cindy's sex life and they had no secrets. Cindy proceeded to tell me in excruciating detail about her promiscuous behavior. She was unhappy with the side effects of the birth control pills (she had a bad case of acne, weight gain, and fatigue, and her periods all but disappeared) and wanted another option to regulate her periods. She casually remarked that she knew birth control pills didn't help protect her from sexually transmitted diseases, so she was now occasionally using condoms after two episodes of STDs.

I took Cindy off birth control pills and started her on natural progesterone. I also took the opportunity to stress and reinforce that she was not protected from sexually transmitted diseases with the birth control pills or the natural progesterone. We spoke of the great risks she was subjecting herself to through her reckless behavior.

I explained to her mother that her blind support of her daughter was doing more harm than good. Cindy's mother meekly told me she didn't agree with Cindy's lifestyle but thought that by being supportive she would not lose her daughter and maybe Cindy would outgrow this stage of her life faster.

We agreed to discuss how the mother could really help.

The first step was to tell her daughter that she didn't condone her lifestyle. She was afraid her daughter would get angry with her and act out even more, or worse yet, not tell her what she was doing. Unfortunately, while Cindy was telling her mother everything she was doing, her mother didn't take the parental responsibility to guide and set boundaries for her. Out of fear, Cindy's mother failed to confront the dangers associated with Cindy's high-risk lifestyle and truly help her daughter.

Not confronting Cindy could prove deadly. I encouraged her mother to start telling Cindy the truth about how she felt about her life.

Fearful and hesitant at first, Cindy's mother took a few months to confront her daughter. To her surprise, when she finally did— over the minor issue of Cindy going out on a Friday night wearing a tiny tank top—Cindy reacted well. She went back into her bedroom and returned wearing an outfit her mother loved. Feeling reassured by her success, Cindy's mother began addressing her daughter's relationships with boys. Cindy listened.

Meanwhile, on the physiologic front, she had responded nicely to the natural progesterone. Her periods were now more regular, her acne was resolving, and the extra weight was starting to come off.

When I started addressing changes in her diet and the addition of supplements to improve her energy level and help with the weight loss, Cindy cooperated every step of the way. The better she felt, the more cooperative she became.

With her mother's help and her father's reassurance that she was beautiful and didn't need to be promiscuous to be popular, she slowly changed her ways.

Today she has one boyfriend, and she wears makeup only on special occasions. I must admit Cindy was an easy teen to work with because she had supportive and cooperative parents. Sometimes the resolution of the teen identity problem is not as smooth or as successful. Family interactions are often difficult, and parental support is not as easy to come by. I try to work with the parents and the teen to find common ground, because I often find that both sides want to help and be helped but don't know how to get together.

"We just keep on doing it until we get it right" is Monica's motto. She has been working with her daughter Marlene for six years, and although things are smoother now, she believes her work as a parent will never be done. I agree with her whole-heartedly. "That's life. I'd never have it any other way," Monica says.

At twelve, Marlene was a pudgy, insulin-resistant, acne-covered, moody young kid whom no one wanted to be around. Her mother and I worked endlessly to provide guidance, support, and treatment for Marlene. And there were many times when we hit our heads against a solid brick wall. Marlene refused to follow a junk-food-free diet. She didn't want to stop drinking soda or start drinking water. When she felt so sick she could not go to school, Monica used the opportunity to feed her high-protein meals and hydrate her with water and green tea. When Marlene refused to take her natural progesterone and her periods and acne became intolerable, her mother brought the progesterone to her bedroom before bedtime and sat with her until she took it.

When Marlene felt better, her mother made her aware of the connection between the hormones and diet changes and the improvement in her condition.

Marlene was in trouble in school, at home, everywhere she turned. She lied and cheated, she even stole. Her mother never gave up. She gently and kindly confronted Marlene every time she got into trouble. She asked her why she stole, lied, or cheated. Even if the answer was a cascade of excuses, insults, or blaming others, her mother never wavered. She wanted to know why, and she would not take anything less than the truth for an answer.

She wanted Marlene to become responsible for her actions.

In time Marlene began to realize that her life was a reflection and direct outcome of her own behavior. She ran out of excuses. Her mother set the example of honesty and accountability, and Marlene had no choice but to follow in her mother's footsteps.

Today Marlene is a college freshman. Her face has cleared up, her periods are still irregular on occasion, and she has no weight problem or insulin-resistance. She is polite, kind, respectful, and helpful to all.

Marlene is the perfect example of the light at the end of the tunnel. There are times when that light looks awfully dim, though.

Bonnie was fifteen when she was diagnosed with borderline personality disorder. Her parents were devastated. Bonnie had been a regular preteen. She did relatively well in school and had a few friends. Her parents had no reason to expect trouble ahead. There was no family history of mental illness or problems with socialization.

When Bonnie turned eleven, she started to menstruate. Her periods started out regular, and she sailed through the following two years without problems. Then something started to change. She started to have irregular periods. Sometimes she had a period every month, and other times she'd go for twelve weeks without a period. During the months without a period she started to gain weight and her personality changed.

At first she became unreliable. If she stopped to see a friend after school or went out for a slice of pizza, she usually called to tell her mother. Suddenly she stopped. Hours would pass, and her mother wouldn't know what had happened to Bonnie. At first her mother became angry and yelled at Bonnie when she finally came home. That reaction only angered Bonnie, who didn't seem to care and became even more troubled.

Later her mother started to punish her. She had read a book

on tough love and decided this was the only way to straighten Bonnie out. The more she was punished, the worse Bonnie behaved.

It all came to a head on a Friday night when Bonnie went out to visit a friend and didn't return for two days. Her mother reported her missing and spent two days crying, sure that something horrible had happened to her child. When she returned, Bonnie calmly said that she had been at a friend's house the whole time and didn't understand what the big deal was. Her mother said Bonnie was old enough to know better, and Bonnie told her mother to just "butt out of my life."

Things went from bad to worse. Bonnie's moods became a minefield, her weight skyrocketed, and she started to smoke cigarettes and marijuana. One second she was fine, nice, pleasant and sweet, and the next she was a monster, as though an alien entered her mind and vile words came rushing out of her mouth. Her friends and family were mortified.

Bonnie's bad behavior was not limited to her parents but affected her peer group as well. Her old friends started avoiding her, and she made new friends among kids whose interests lay far away from education and family.

Bonnie's pediatrician recommended psychiatric help. Her mother wanted to know about help with her diet, but the doctor thought that the diet should wait, that her personality problem was more pressing. The psychiatrist diagnosed Bonnie with borderline personality disorder and placed her on medication to balance her mood swings.

She improved a little, but the following four years were a nightmare. The medication worsened her weight problem and affected her hormone balance, which translated into irregular periods and serious acne.

I saw Bonnie at the psychiatrist's recommendation. He believed her hormones were out of balance even though her blood tests showed normal hormone levels. He requested a second opinion from me.

I don't like medical diagnostic labels because I believe they affect long-term outcome. Diagnoses like borderline personality disorder are damaging to both the patient and the family. I believe they hinder improvement or resolution of the condition. I prefer simple descriptions, like "problems with teen behavior." Problems have solutions and can be solved.

When I saw Bonnie, I didn't see a patient with borderline personality disorder. I saw yet another troubled teen. Her problems had started at the age of thirteen, two years after she got her period. It was at this time that her periods became irregular, she started gaining weight, and her moods became unmanageable.

With the knowledge we now have of how the teen's body functions, it was clear the problems were hormone-related. Unfortunately, this now-obvious root cause for the sudden transformation in Bonnie was overlooked in her diagnosis and treatment plan, and the entire focus was placed on the behavioral problems. The family and child had now suffered for years without reprieve or hope for a solution in sight.

When I saw Bonnie, I treated her with natural progesterone, 200 milligrams a day in cream form, for the whole month, stopping when her period started, and I placed her on the basic supplements: L-carnitine, coenzyme Q_{10}, and omega-3 (see chapter 3).

I met with Bonnie alone and together with her parents. The communication lines were closed. No one spoke. The family was so traumatized by Bonnie's behavior that they walked on eggshells around her.

She was considered ill and was treated as such.

My approach to Bonnie was to establish one ground rule: while she was under my care, the whole family had to forget Bonnie's psychiatric diagnosis. Then we could treat her just like another misbehaving teen.

My approach worked. Bonnie was off medications within six months, and her behavior returned to tolerable.

Solutions

- I started Bonnie on 200 milligrams of natural progesterone in cream form for the whole month. She stopped only when she got her period.
- I started Bonnie on supplements (Dr. Erika's Essential Elements for Teens—see chapter 3).
- We limited the amount of junk food and soda in her diet.
- Bonnie and her mother agreed that she would be treated like an adult only if she acted like one.
- We started a responsibility/reward system:

  - If Bonnie called when she was going to be late, she would be allowed to go out more frequently.
  - If Bonnie cleaned her room, she would be rewarded with a reasonable perk of her choice (e.g., going to a movie or a friend's house).
  - If Bonnie addressed her parents politely, they would respond positively and reinforce her behavior.
  - Negatives would be kept to a minimum. I instructed the parents to never mention the old diagnosis or equate any of Bonnie's bad behavior with her being sick or handicapped. (If she did

something wrong, the problem would be addressed but not linked to previous episodes of problems.)

- Bonnie had to be treated like a normal person. No one is perfect, and Bonnie's family learned to treat her like everyone else.

Within two months, Bonnie was more reliable, and working with her became an increasingly pleasant task. Her parents were reassured, and as her behavior improved—with the help of the new tools we were using (natural progesterone, supplements, dietary changes, behavior modification)—the family became more relaxed and optimistic.

Along with this improvement they decided to allow Bonnie to switch schools. At the new school Bonnie did not carry the label of her old diagnosis and became integrated remarkably well in a short time. No longer an outcast, she became part of her peer group community, and this time she chose a group that matched her newfound self-image.

Bonnie's story is not unusual. I see many troubled teens with serious diagnoses of behavioral problems improve almost miraculously with my integrated program of natural hormones, supplements, dietary adjustments, and behavioral guidelines.

How to Help Your Teen Handle Peer Pressure

At the age of thirteen, Karen decided her parents were too uneducated for her and moved in with one of her friends from school. Her parents were devastated but could not convince Karen to come back home.

Karen was attending a parochial school, and her parents were factory workers. Her peer group was made up of children of parents with higher education and greater means.

I met Karen's mother at a lecture I was giving at a women's club in her town in Illinois. Her mother approached me at the end of the lecture and asked for guidance. I was spending two days in their town, so I agreed to meet over tea the next morning. Her story was heart-wrenching.

She and her husband had five children. They both worked two jobs in two factories to put food on the table and give their children what they themselves didn't have growing up. Karen was the third child and the brightest. The only problem Karen had was her weight, which she blamed on her parents. It was true that their diet consisted of a lot of junk food. Karen's parents understood that their diet was not the best but felt that in time the weight would come off and Karen would be happy.

They sent her to private school to give her a better chance at higher education. And the child left them. Karen's mother had tears in her eyes.

I suggested that Karen call me, and I gave her mom my cell phone number. To my surprise, she did call. She was hesitant but willing to talk. She told me she was embarrassed by her parents and her home, and the only solution she saw was to move out and live among the people she wanted to be like. She also stated that her new family ate good foods and believed in exercise. She wanted to be like them.

I asked Karen if she cared for her parents and if she understood that it was through their sacrifice that she had access to the peer group she emulated. She said she knew it but felt she had no options. The only way she saw to lose weight and be accepted was to leave her family. She asked if I could explain this to her mother.

I had a better idea. I suggested Karen do the explaining.

My advice for Karen was to go home and make dinner for her family the following weekend. Without leaving her peer group, I hoped she could start bridging the gap and bringing her new-found knowledge of diet and health to her family. I was certain Karen's mother would never get in the way of Karen's perceived advancement in the world. I strongly believed that Karen needed to integrate her family and peer group.

If Karen's friends did not support her connection to her family, they were not real friends. Karen needed to understand that she was a combination of her original family and her friends. Living without either group, she would be incomplete. She needed to take the best from both worlds and bring them together.

I get a Christmas card from Karen every year. She is now in college, and she goes home to her parents for the holidays. She has made her family proud, her weight is no longer a problem, and in turn her family is no longer living on junk food alone.

Peer pressure is a powerful influence in our teens' lives. Short of keeping them locked up in the house, we cannot prevent their friends from affecting their lives.

The advice I give my patients and my own teens is the following:

- Be realistic about what your teen is about. Do not deny the existence of the problem.
- Be honest with your teen. Tell her what you think about her friends without being unkind or hurtful.

- Do not expect your teen to listen to you and give up a friend just because you tell her you know the friend is not a real friend.
- Wait it out. If you are correct and do not make things difficult, in time your teen may come around.
- Help your teen become aware and realistic about her relationships with her peers. Do not condone abusive behavior.

How to Raise a Well-Balanced, Socially Aware, and Adept Teen

After you get your teen's hormones in balance, her weight as close to ideal as realistically possible, and her moods in reasonable check, you still have a job to perform as a parent. As a physician and parent myself, I find the following basic guidelines important to follow to complete the picture that we call success:

- *Don't be afraid of your teen.* Fear is dangerous. If you are afraid, she will act out more.
- *Listen to your teen.* Help her figure out who she really is. She isn't a mini-version of you or your ideals.
- *Acknowledge the importance of her complaints.* If she isn't happy, there is a reason for it. Help her figure out the real reason. You might not agree with the reason, but you must respect its validity if you are committed to helping her.
- *Be honest about your teen.* Do not sweep the problems under the rug hoping they will disappear. Do not justify her poor behavior.

- *Develop trust.* If she believes you respect her and acknowledge her issues and find them valid, she will start speaking to you. It might take months to get there, even years, but it will happen and the wait is well worth it.

- *Set up a system that encourages her to work with you to solve the problem.* If she feels listened to and validated, she will work with you.

- *Define the limits and be flexible with them.* This is not the time to win a popularity contest with your teen. If you do it right, you will become her hero by the time she finishes college.

- *Be responsible and expect responsibility in return.* Practice what you preach. If you make plans, keep them. Stay in touch, call frequently, and keep her abreast of your whereabouts if you want your teen to do the same.

- *Be kind and expect kindness in return.* Teens are very sensitive and insecure. The slightest criticism will be misinterpreted. Do not walk around on eggshells, do not avoid telling the truth. Do it kindly and not judgmentally. She needs your input to survive the harsh outside world.

- *Set a good example and you will get a great teen.* If you make every effort to be decent, honest, and kind, your teen will follow. You have the wisdom of experience, and if you impart that knowledge to your teen in the proper form, she will listen.

- *Let her see you as you are, not an idealized version.* We are all human, and adults are full of flaws. While I don't encourage you to start drinking in front of your teen, I do encourage you to be honest about your mistakes and struggles. She needs your strength, but above all, she needs you to be real.

- *Be patient!* In time, everything works out. You always have another day to make it better. Nothing is lost if today was a bust. You can make tomorrow a success!

7

Diet, Body Image, and Exercise

Whether adult or teen, most of us are constantly deciding to lose weight by going on a diet. For adults, dieting is a conscious and often desperate exercise. For teens, it is a combination of lip service and occasionally successful honest attempts.

Inevitably, though, even if the weight does come off for a while, it reappears as soon as we stop the diet and go back to our old eating and living habits.

Diets fail because:

1. Your hormones are not in balance.
2. The diet is inappropriate for you in particular.
3. You don't follow it correctly.
4. Nothing has changed when you go back to your old habits after the dieting is over.

While the second, third, and fourth reasons are common knowledge, the first is a critical factor that is mostly overlooked and poorly understood.

Having read this book this far, you are now aware of the unavoidable connection between your adolescent's weight gain and the state of her hormone balance. The next step is to realize that if your teen or you are not losing weight while following a diet, you need to look for other symptoms of hormone imbalance, then treat the problem and balance the hormones.

To get this crucial message out, I needed to work out the details of a plan that incorporates hormone balancing with diets in my own practice.

I work with a number of nutritionists who refer their teen clients to me when diets alone are not the answer. The opportunity to work with teens who have failed to lose weight through diets alone proved an eye-opener to me. Through my experience with these teens, I have been able to prove the hormone balance connection. If I could start or speed up the rate of weight loss in teens with weight problems by balancing their hormones, I could potentially solve most weight problems for teens.

Working with the nutritionists, I established the following process for the teens they referred to me:

1. Identify teens who are not doing as well as expected on diet and nutritionally supervised weight reduction programs.
2. Determine if they have other symptoms of hormone imbalance that would reinforce the possibility that hormones are the root cause of their problem: acne,

    irregular periods, insulin-resistance, diagnosis of PCOs, mood swings, severe PMS, cramps, or headaches.

3. Have these teens evaluated by their personal physician with blood tests to eliminate the presence of other medical problems.

4. Once completing the first three steps, start them on natural progesterone and supplements to balance their hormones and increase metabolism by increasing energy production.

5. Finally, have the teens followed by the nutritionist and measure weight loss after starting hormone and supplements therapy.

I applied similar principles when reestablishing hormone balance in adult women with natural hormones, with remarkably positive results. My methods and program are published in *The Hormone Solution* and *The 30-Day Natural Hormone Plan*. Although I initially made the hormone connection with menopausal women, the books are not limited to that age group; the information connecting hormones with symptoms are applicable to men and women of all ages.

Teens and Diet

With the growing problem of teen obesity, I started to see more teens. The problems with them were a little different from adult problems with obesity: teen follow-through on anything, let alone diet, is a difficult challenge, and problems with their hormone balance are not addressed head-on in our medical culture.

My resounding success with the teens' mothers started to

change the configuration of my practice. The connection between balancing their hormones and successfully losing weight became an impetus for mothers to bring in their overweight teens.

This is how the combination of natural hormones, their balance and diet came together successfully for the teens I treat.

What Options Do Overweight Teens Have?

Overweight teens have no place to go in conventional medicine.

Unless they are diagnosed with insulin-resistance or polycystic ovary syndrome, the role of hormone imbalance in teen obesity isn't addressed by our conventional medical system.

The scientific literature confirms the direct connection between obesity and hormone imbalance in teens but doesn't propose correcting the presumed hormone imbalances as a first line of treatment.

To make a difficult situation even harder, success is measured in terms of numbers of pounds lost, not overall improvement in physical and mental state.

Gail was sixteen when her mother took her to the pediatrician to have her hormones checked. She had gained twenty pounds in the previous year, had acne, and had irregular periods. Gail was a great girl. She did well in school and never complained about her weight, or anything else for that matter. Gail's mother, on the other hand, became increasingly worried about Gail's weight problem and took action.

The pediatrician recommended an endocrinologist, who sent Gail for a battery of blood tests and then diagnosed her with high testosterone levels and insulin-resistance. Devastated, Gail's mother found a center for endocrine disorders and weight loss in their town in Pennsylvania and immediately enrolled Gail in their program.

The first time Gail went to the center, her mother went along. The girls in the group were all very obese. Gail felt out of place, and her mother knew this wasn't the right place for her.

They came to see me. Gail's mother was looking for help with weight loss. Gail was just scared that something was wrong with her.

By now you know what I recommended:

- Natural progesterone to improve her hormone balance, regulate her periods, and help her feel better fast
- Supplements to enhance her metabolic energy production, hormone manufacture, and sense of well-being
- Dietary adjustments, including limitation of fast foods, soda, and junk food.
- Increased water intake to help flush out toxins and clear the system
- Stress management to decrease the impact of stressors in Gail's life

The results were remarkable. Gail felt better in less than a month. Her skin cleared, she felt more energetic, and she was no longer scared that something was terribly wrong with her.

We were left with two issues after two months: she had lost only two pounds, and she was still wearing baggy clothes to conceal her weight. In the next few pages, I will show you how we solved these two problems as well.

Girls and Their Bodies

Numerous pop psychology books have been written about girls and their body image, transformation, and the changes that occur throughout adolescence. These books focus on the psychology of the change, the problems associated with the transition from child to adult woman, and the stumbling blocks our society throws in the way of making the transition smooth.

During adolescence, lean body mass increases. The increase is greater in males because they develop more muscle mass as their hormones are activated. Girls, however, start depositing fat throughout puberty. This normal process is the physiologic way the female body is built. Without this fat deposition, girls would never menstruate or become fertile.

Unfortunately, as our society heads toward rising obesity rates and cultural difficulties with calibrating body image, the natural transition from girl to woman is becoming less clear-cut.

Obesity and Puberty

In the following few paragraphs, I address issues related to obese teens. Overweight teens are not obese teens. In the introduction, I described in detail how weight is measured and statistically quantified in clinical medicine. The formulas and graphs are often confusing and difficult to follow. The definition of obesity is often vague, and the impact of the term "obesity" is traumatic and pejorative. Personally and professionally, I hesitate to use it. I am using it here solely in the context of information used by your physician. The point of conveying this information is to reinforce the hormonal component of weight problems.

1. Obese female adolescents tend toward earlier sexual maturation and start menstruating at a younger age.

2. Owing to pituitary-hypothalamic (the master glands in the brain that control hormone release and balance) changes in obese girls, hormone production and transformation take different paths. Increased production of testosterone and its transformation into estrogen creates irregular, heavy periods in obese teens.

3. Five percent of obese children actually carry a diagnosis of an endocrine (hormone) problem.

4. Genetic factors have been found to significantly influence chances for obesity in teens. In a Swedish twins study, if one parent was obese, the risk was 30 percent for the child to become obese. If both parents were obese, the risk rose to 50 percent.

5. Despite the genetic factor theory, environmental and cultural factors are of significant importance.

Eating Disorders:
Hormonal and Emotional Influences

Millicent was diagnosed with a combination eating disorder—anorexia and bulimia. I saw her because her mother was convinced that Millicent's problems were hormone-related and that the psychiatric care she was receiving was not enough to help her.

Millicent started menstruating at the age of twelve and a half. She had been a picky eater as a child, and when she entered puberty she was very thin. Apparently Millicent liked being very thin, and she wasn't happy with the way her body started to change when she entered puberty. As a result, she stopped eating, hoping her breasts would stop growing and her body stop becoming more womanly.

She was only partially successful. At fourteen, she was five-foot-two and weighed less than ninety pounds. Her period disappeared, and she was diagnosed with anorexia, placed in intensive psychotherapy, and put on medication. She was also seeing a nutritionist and an adolescent medicine specialist.

With the help of medication, her parents, and the whole medical team, Millicent gained weight over the following year and stabilized at 102 pounds. Her period returned. With it also came the physical changes she had dreaded so much at twelve. Her breasts grew, and she started to look like a young woman.

She didn't like the changes at all. This time, though, she found a new way to conceal the physical appearance she disliked. She started to binge. Within a period of six months, she gained twenty-five pounds, and with her tiny frame she looked seriously overweight. Confused about her body image, Millicent began to alternate periods of bingeing with periods of total anorexia. Her entire life was focused on her dangerous eating habits.

The therapists focused on her eating disorder, and Millicent focused on her eating disorder. Then I was called in to help.

When I first saw Millicent, I was struck by the fact that she was lost in her eating disorder. She told me that her insides were always shaking and she was obsessing about food to the exclusion of everything else in her life. It was the best way to avoid what really bothered her, which was that she didn't want to grow up and be a woman.

Her mother was correct: the problem needed addressing from both the hormone and psychological standpoints. If Millicent's hormones hadn't started to function, she wouldn't have had to contend with the physical changes she feared. Her eating disorder might not have developed at all. Unfortunately for Millicent, Mother Nature has her plan, and normal healthy teens do not escape puberty.

Millicent needed help accepting reality and some hormonal support for a smoother transition into adolescence.

I started Millicent on natural progesterone (200 milligrams in cream form) every evening for two months. She needed progesterone because her periods had been so irregular that she was unlikely to ovulate, and without ovulation her body wasn't making enough progesterone to balance her. The symptoms of anxiety manifested by the butterflies in her stomach also led me to think that she would benefit from additional progesterone. To my relief and reassurance, Millicent felt calmer within a week. She said her insides had stopped shaking.

Shortly thereafter, she stopped bingeing and throwing up. Her therapist told me that she felt she could get through to Millicent more easily.

Within six months' time, Millicent had stopped taking medication, become interested in socializing, and joined the yearbook staff at school. By the time she turned seventeen, she was helping other girls with eating disorders identify hormone problems as core issues and referring them to me for treatment.

How Your Eating Habits Affect Your Teens

Dina, a forty-nine-year-old successful investment banker, brought her daughter Martha to see me. She was concerned that Martha had an eating disorder.

Sixteen-year-old Martha was five feet tall, weighed ninety-two pounds, and immediately upon meeting me informed me that she believed she had an eating disorder. The history was interesting and not unusual.

Dina was beautiful and very health-conscious. She ate only macrobiotic foods, worked out with a trainer four times a week, and spared no time or expense on looking and feeling young.

Martha was growing up in this environment. She too was now obsessed with every calorie that entered her mouth and every minute she spent on the treadmill. Her weight had never been a problem until the breakup with her boyfriend three months before. While recovering, she found herself eating less and exercising more. She shared that information with her mother, who immediately took her to a nutritionist. The nutritionist addressed the diet issue and prescribed an increase in protein and complex carbohydrates. The nutritionist told Martha that this diet would help her increase muscle mass and would not make her gain weight.

When Martha came home and told her mother the nutritionist's advice, Dina immediately jumped on the bandwagon and decided to go on the same diet with Martha. Martha was unhappy and felt abandoned. She believed she had an eating disorder, and her mother, instead of acting like the parent, was trying to emulate her problem.

I saw Martha alone for a few visits. We spoke of her conflict about being like her mother and trying to be different. Martha liked the way her mother looked and took care of herself, but she wanted to have her own identity. Moreover, she didn't want her mother to copy her, even though she was copying her mother. Her vacillation stemmed from being unclear about her body image and identity.

I saw Dina twice and gave her the following advice. She had failed to see the similarity between her obsession with weight and her daughter's and needed to acknowledge her daughter's concern with having an eating disorder. In other words, Dina needed to become a mother and not a pal to Martha. That meant providing her daughter with encouragement, guidance, and support. Dina also had to acknowledge her own problems with weight and body image as a source for Martha's problems. Both Dina and Martha had to be honest with each other and address the striking similarities in their problems.

Together they did well. They started to talk about the problems they both had with body image and their shared obsessive need to be thin. In time Martha understood that she was separate from her mother, and she went on to college, where she adjusted well and did not have eating problems again.

Realistic Nutritional Goals for Teens

To keep your teen healthy and free of weight problems, we need to look at how guidelines for nutritional supplementation are created and what they measure. Although the terms are dry and difficult to comprehend, they serve the basic purpose of providing a standardized means of looking at the nutritional values of our foods.

They provide the criteria for supplementation in teens that your doctors and nutritionists will be using. Being familiar with them will make your life easier and any encounter with the health-care field or supermarket food labels less onerous.

1. Recommended dietary allowance (RDA): This is the amount of particular nutrients almost all healthy individuals need to maintain health. Among healthy

people in North America, 98 to 99 percent eat this amount of nutrients in their regular diet.

2. Adequate intake (AI): When RDA cannot be determined, AI is a value based on experimental or observational approximations. Adequate intake is an amount of a nutrient that is enough to keep a person from being undernourished.

3. Estimated average requirement (EAR): The EAR is the estimated requirement to meet a need for a particular nutrient.

4. Tolerable upper intake level (TUL): This is the maximum level of intake of a daily nutrient that is unlikely to create adverse effects in almost all the individuals in the group for which it is designed (for instance, the largest amount of a vitamin the average person most likely to take that vitamin can take without developing side effects).

When reading the label on a nutritional supplement, you may encounter one or more of the above nutritional requirement criteria. This does not imply that you should rely solely on these values to determine your teen's appropriate diet balance. The reality is that you need to figure out how to balance your teen's food intake to create a healthy internal environment. To achieve success in this area, your teen needs energy.

Energy is derived from the foods we eat. Determined by growth needs and level of activity, energy is measured in calories. Calories represent the result of the transformation of foods into energy. The higher the caloric content, the more energy the food can potentially generate.

Now you are thinking: a cheeseburger with French fries should be an ideal meal. It certainly has lots of calories. Unfortunately for all you fast-food lovers out there, this is not at all an ideal meal. Most of the energy created from the breakdown of fast foods gets wasted in the process.

The process of making energy involves chemical reactions conducted in the cells under the supervision of hormones. All foods need energy to break them down, but fast foods create enormous amounts of toxic waste during the breakdown process. Cleaning up the toxic wastes at the cellular level where energy is made also takes a lot of energy. The result is that more energy is wasted cleaning up after a junk food meal than is generated to use in important cellular reactions. A perfect example is hormone production. We need lots of energy to make hormones and keep them in balance. If our cells are busy cleaning up after junk food meals, they don't have time or energy to cater to our hormone needs. As a result, the hormone balance is thrown off, and within a short few hours after eating a hamburger and French fries, your teen is exhausted and has essentially no energy.

We desperately need to help our teens eat the right foods.

Samantha was a twelve-year-old star athlete. She was the captain of her soccer team and a performance skier. Her parents brought her to me because she was constantly fatigued. She ate regular meals, and her coach gave her candy bars before each practice and game. She slept well and was a good student. She had not gotten her period yet, and her pediatrician told the family that this was normal: her period was delayed because of her high level of physical activity and low body fat content. No one worried about the period, but all were concerned about her constant state of fatigue.

Samantha was a perfect example of poor eating habits. Although from a distance she appeared to be eating well-balanced meals, a closer look revealed a different story. The regular meals she ate, while high in protein, did not contain enough complex carbohydrates, and the candy bars her coach gave her drained her energy even more. You may recall that processed carbohydrates, which candy bars are made of, are rapidly absorbed into the bloodstream and raise the blood sugar level temporarily. Insulin quickly comes into the picture and pushes all the sugar into the cells, leaving the candy bar eater with lower blood sugar than she started with and drained of energy to boot.

Teens and athletes need continuous fueling to keep their energy-making factories well stoked. The best fuel is a combination of carbohydrates and protein that comes from frequent meals and unprocessed foods.

Eating every three hours is important for growing bodies, especially teens with rapidly changing hormones who are also athletic. We feed our babies every three to four hours, and then we teach our aging adults to eat frequent meals.

We need to teach our teens the importance of eating frequent meals as well.

Samantha went on a regular diet high in protein and complex carbohydrates, eating every three hours, and her energy improved remarkably. I also added supplements to her regimen: omega-3 fatty acids to increase her good fat content, and L-carnitine and coenzyme Q_{10} to stoke her energy-making cellular factories.

What Foods Should Your Teen Be Eating?

FATS

The caloric content of fats is the highest of all foods. That makes them a great source of energy. Fatty acids—the small molecules that fat is broken down into by the time it gets into the blood-stream—are the building blocks of hormones. The better the fats, the more effective the hormone production assembly line.

Fats are essential to your teen's hormone balance, and knowing how to make the distinction between good and bad fats is critical to proper nutrition and efficient energy production.

Good Fats

- Fish oils, known as omega-3 DHA (docosahexaenoic acid) and EPA (ethyl-eicosapentaenoate); found in most cold-water and deep-ocean fish, such as halibut, cod, salmon, tuna, sardines, and mackerel
- Flaxseed oil, also known as omega-6 linoleic and linolenic acids; found in green leafy vegetables and safflower, borage, and evening primrose oils
- Olive oil—cold-pressed and virgin.

Good fats are very important to your teen's well-being. They help with their moods, stabilize their hormone balance, make their hair shine and their nails strong, and even improve their complexion.

Bad Fats

- Trans-fatty acids, found in margarine and butter substitutes
- Chemically developed synthetic fat substitutes; identifiable by their chemical taste and found in all preserved foods (not in fresh foods)

Animal Fats

These are fats that come from animal sources and when used in moderation will give your teen energy but may over time add weight and cause hormone imbalance. The best advice is to eat them no more than once a week.

- Bacon
- Butter
- Sour cream
- Fat on meats (fatty parts of steak, pork chops, skin on poultry, yellow fat globules in chicken and beef soups)

A FEW WORDS ABOUT CHOLESTEROL

With the growing epidemic of overweight teens, physicians are starting to see more teens with high cholesterol levels than ever before.

Cholesterol is a complex fat. It is an important substance, and its effects are not all negative. Cholesterol is an integral component of hormone production and brain function. There is both good and bad cholesterol. Good cholesterol HDL is a key ingredient in hormone production and is high in physically active teens. You want to encourage your teen to work out and thus increase good cholesterol. It helps with the way she looks and her hormone balance as well. Bad cholesterol, LDL, is at the root of the deposits in our arteries and the premature aging we are now finding in our teens on high-fat diets. LDL is found in processed foods and trans-fatty acids in junk food like potato chips, cookies, and other junk snacks.

The ideal situation is to provide a well-balanced diet for your teen that includes enough healthy fats for her body to be able to manufacture the needed amounts of cholesterol for hormone production and not raise cholesterol to abnormal levels.

Teens should not have to go on low-cholesterol diets or take medication to lower their cholesterol levels. Starting them on healthy diets and teaching them to stay away from saturated fats and junk food should prove enough.

SUGARS

Also known as carbs or carbohydrates, sugars come in many forms. Confusion about sugars abounds. We cannot live without sugars. Glucose is the basic sugar our bodies use to make and store energy. Insulin is the hormone that recognizes and responds to blood glucose levels (not the amount of cake or candy you've eaten). Desserts, ice cream, all things sweet, contain glucose. It is the glucose molecule that goes into our bloodstream after we digest all our sweets that produces an increase in our blood sugar levels. Our body uses glucose molecules to make energy. Chemical reactions in every cell in the body transform glucose molecules into energy.

So why aren't sweets great for our teens?

Because most sweets contain highly processed and refined carbohydrates. They may taste good, but just like the cheeseburger, instead of building your teen's energy stores, these foods bog them down with toxic waste and wear them down.

The refined carbs found in sweets, candy bars, the ubiquitous corn syrup, and other junk foods get absorbed very quickly into the bloodstream (like the hamburger and French fries). The result is a rapid rise in blood glucose levels. This triggers insulin production that pushes the sugar into the cells leading to hypoglycemia, and leaves the teen drained and stressed. Another hormone you may remember that plays a role in the constant roller coaster of fast foods is cortisol, which rises whenever insulin levels rise and wears down the brain and every other organ, leaving behind a drained teen. And all sugar that is stored from the breakdown of the sweets is turned into fat cells, leading to the worst-case scenario: apparently unavoidable weight gain.

PROTEINS

Critical to hormone production and the maintenance of body weight, proteins come from two sources: animal and vegetable. Although vegetables do contain a fair amount of protein, teens who are vegetarian often run into trouble with low-protein intake. To get enough protein into the body, especially the growing body of a teen, we need animal proteins. Unless your teen is philosophically opposed to animal sources for protein, I believe animal-source protein is an integral part of a complete diet for a healthy teen.

Adding protein concentrates to the diet of a teen is a source of debate among nutritionists. While protein supplementation for adults is routine today, adding protein to teens' diets is not always necessary. Unless the teen is suffering from protein deficiency syndromes (loss of muscle mass, intestinal problems, foggy thinking, loss of hair sheen, thinning nails), a well-balanced diet should provide enough protein.

Teens who are athletes and body builders will benefit from protein additives without hormones, but the average teen who is fighting a weight problem and trying to balance her hormones need not worry about protein supplementation.

Vegetable-Source Protein

- Beans
- Nuts
- Soy
- Yams

Animal-Source Protein

- All animal meats: poultry beef, pork, etc.
- Dairy: milk, cheese, yogurt, buttermilk, eggs, sour cream

Fish-Source Protein

- All fish meats: tuna, salmon, cod, swordfish, sardines, striped bass, etc.

- All shellfish: lobster, shrimp, clams, mussels, oysters, octopus, squid, scallops, crabs

All these sources of protein, once broken down into their basic molecules (called amino acids), enter the bloodstream and are used to make hormones, muscles, bones, tendons, and cartilage and help maintain your teen's brain power and physical growth. The ideal balance of hormones and weight is maintained with the proper intake of protein in balance with fats, carbohydrates, and fiber.

FIBER

I am sure you've been hearing about fiber for years. I find it surprising that when I ask people what fiber is, they don't know.

Fiber is not the same as starches, even though many of the starches contain fiber. Fiber has always been part of our diet, but it was only about fifteen years ago that it became its own category. Fiber is very important to your teen because it can balance the negative effects of high insulin and help maintain hormone balance while also being of help with weight control.

To explain why fiber is so important, we have to once again turn to our old friend insulin. Remember, constant insulin spikes erode your teen's body and every internal organ from heart to brain to kidney. The only way to stop insulin from spiking is to maintain a constant blood sugar level that keeps insulin levels even as well.

Fiber helps contain and control insulin and sugar spikes. Fiber works in a very complex way. It is almost indigestible. Unlike fats, sugars, or proteins, it cannot be broken down into small molecules. Large fiber molecules just float around our system. Fiber doesn't provide the teen's body with nutrients either, nor is it digested. Yet, by its sheer existence, fiber prevents other foods from being rapidly absorbed into the bloodstream and thus slows down the rise of blood sugar in the bloodstream. In turn, insulin levels don't rise because sugar levels are even.

So why don't we just eat a lot of fiber? Why don't we make all our foods full of fiber and feed them to our teens? The problem is that fiber is difficult to tolerate. Our stomach and intestines quickly get bloated if we eat too much fiber. Our teens have taste buds that are already used to eating junk, so fiber is a learned pleasure. Only when they realize how much better they feel when they eat fiber will our teens eat more of it.

In the appendix are family dinner menus. They contain a good balance of the important nutritional elements we have just addressed. Use them to train your teen's palate to become accustomed to eating more fiber.

Fiber-Rich Foods

- Apples
- Asparagus
- Berries
- Bok choy (Chinese cabbage)
- Bran
- Broccoli
- Broccoli rabe
- Brussels sprouts
- Cabbages—any type
- Cauliflower
- Collard greens
- Cucumbers
- Eggplant
- Garlic
- Grits

- Kale
- Lettuce (any type)
- Oats and oatmeal
- Onions
- Peas
- Peppers
- Radishes
- Spinach
- String beans
- Turnips
- Watercress
- Zucchini

Follow the menus in the appendix and create a social dinner atmosphere where food is not the focus but rather the vehicle to a healthy introduction for your teen to her adult life. Your teen uses you as a role model regardless of what she says. The apple doesn't fall far from the tree!

Make life your focus, not food and weight!

8

Teen Rebellion

One method of research I used in preparation for this book was a series of interviews I conducted with both teens and mothers of teens. For this particular chapter, I spoke with twenty mothers and their daughters and ten teens alone.

Many of the questions I asked were related to lifestyle because I strongly believe the weight problem in teens (or adults) will not be solved unless we have a complete picture (as much as possible) of the person in need of treatment. The only way I can resolve the weight problem is to understand how the particular teen's life and her environment influence her weight.

My goal in writing this book is to help as many teens and their families as possible to find long-term solutions for the growing weight problem. The connection between lifestyle, teen behavior, and weight are sidebars addressed in most weight-loss programs, which focus instead on The Diet!

Once the lifestyle connection is made by both the clinician try-ing to help and the teen and her support system (in this case her mother), providing individually helpful tools to reduce or even eliminate the weight problem raises the chances for success.

I conducted my interviews during consultation sessions or in-dividually at the request of the mother or, rarely, the teen.

If I was successful at integrating as many aspects of the teen's life as possible with the diet and hormone balance problems, and then found support and commitment from the teen and her family to implement all the changes needed, the results were re-markable.

If, however, large obstacles couldn't be overcome (no family support was available, the teen wouldn't stop noxious habits, the family and/or teen wanted only quick fixes), the results were never quite what we had hoped for.

Reasonable Expectations

I started every interview with the same question: "Tell me what you consider a normal teen." By "normal" I was referring to lifestyle factors—school, family, social behaviors—not asking for ideal weight.

After the initial "I don't know" answer, the teens unanimously agreed that "normal" was anything and everything teen. Any-thing the teen's peer group considered *in* ("cool," for those of us from the 1970s and 1980s) was considered normal: teen dress, lifestyles, diets, getting along with parents or not, participating in sports, music, school performance, watching MTV and reality shows, helping around the house, going on family vacations, hav-ing annual physicals, taking vitamins—essentially everything the group endorsed.

If you were a lucky parent of a teen who belonged to a peer group that did everything you hoped your teen would do, you were basically home free. Unfortunately, most teens don't make their parents' lives that easy.

On the other hand, the mothers' responses were not unanimous. There were three dominant opinions of what made for a normal teen.

A small but surprising number of mothers considered a "normal" teen a kind of *ideal* teen: one who got along with his/her parents, had no trouble in school, was popular but not too popular, had friends the parents approved of, followed parental advice, was helpful in all house chores, and spent time with the family on her own volition without grumbling. The mothers in this group were determined to *make* their teen behave in these ways because they believed they were right and the teen didn't know any better and just had to listen.

A smaller yet significant group of mothers told me that, although they would have liked for their teens to be the ideal teen envisioned by the first group, they considered themselves realists and accepted the peer-pressure factor as crucial to how their teen behaved.

To these mothers normal represented a *compromise* between the teen definition of normal and that of the ideal-seeking parents. This group of mothers invariably expected teens to be polite and to listen to their parents, to have clean-cut dress habits, to perform well at school, and to be involved in sports and other social events. They understood and accepted, however, that music, television, and other lifestyle choices were normally influenced by peer-group preferences.

These mothers compromised to maintain their relationship with their teen, with the goal of maintaining access to the teen so as to be able to guide them and influence their important decisions.

Finally, another small group of mothers accepted teens' behaviors and lifestyles and felt no compelling reason to get involved or offer a diverging opinion. These mothers had a wait-and-see attitude and a fatalistic approach in general: "Che sera, sera," seemed to be their motto.

Armed with this important information about the mothers and daughters I was treating (keep in mind that I treat hormone imbalances and weight problems and am not a therapist), I became determined to help both mothers and myself develop better insights into the teens and find solutions that involved the whole gestalt of their relationships and lifestyles to solve the hormone and weight problems.

Priscilla and Mim are one of the mother-daughter teams I've been working with for the past three years. Priscilla, the mom, is now forty-seven, and Mim is seventeen. I first started seeing Priscilla for hot flashes and insomnia and treated her with a combination of natural hormones and supplements. She also went on my 30-Day Natural Hormone Plan and found great success in our integrative approach to her life.

Satisfied with her personal results, Priscilla brought me her daughter. Mim was fourteen at the time and a bundle of trouble. She was overweight, her periods were irregular, and she suffered with terrible mood swings.

While growing up, Mim had been a great little child. Priscilla didn't have one day of trouble with Mim until three months after she started menstruating at the age of twelve. Within six months of the start of her period, Mim stopped speaking to her parents and blocked the door to her bedroom with a chair at night.

She stopped helping around the house and started doing

poorly in school. She dropped out of after-school activities and spent all her free time watching MTV or hanging out with her friends.

Priscilla didn't approve of Mim's friends. They had multicolored hair and multiple piercings. They weren't good students. Most of them were overweight, and they all went for pizza or McDonald's after school. Priscilla felt that Mim's friends lacked parental supervision in their lives, and she feared that Mim would get into more trouble if she continued to socialize with them.

Mim didn't want to join her family for dinner any longer, and she stopped speaking to her two younger siblings. They weren't cool enough for her.

Priscilla was called into school by the principal, who advised her to place Mim in therapy for her unruly behavior. It was suspected she might be suffering from ADD.

Multiple psychological tests revealed some learning disabilities coupled with behavioral issues. Mim started intensive therapy and was placed on medication. For her irregular periods, she was given birth control pills. The combination of therapies worsened the nightmare for Mim and her family. She gained weight and became even more difficult to manage. With her moods even more unpredictable and her face covered with pimples, Mim was becoming the prototype of the troubled teen.

After two years of acting out and pushing the limits, Priscilla brought Mim to see me out of desperation, hoping her daughter's problems were caused by hormone imbalances. At this point Mim herself was also becoming seriously embarrassed by her weight problem.

Priscilla was right. Mim's problems had started when she began menstruation. The symptoms that followed—irregular periods, mood swings, weight gain—followed the point in time when she started to have her period. They were caused by hormone changes brought on by the beginning of puberty and followed by the onset of menstruation.

The treatments and evaluations she underwent addressed primarily Mim's behavior problems, and the birth control pills didn't balance her hormones—in fact, they overrode her system and even possibly worsened her hormone imbalances and moods.

By addressing her hormone problems, I knew I could help improve the whole picture of Mim's troubled teen life. I began by advising Mim to stop taking birth control pills. She did so without hesitation. She was sexually active and told me she knew birth control pills did not protect her from sexually transmitted diseases so she was using condoms faithfully.

Next, Mim and her mother agreed to jointly keep a journal of what they ate. Priscilla was already on the 30-Day Natural Hormone Plan and so she knew how to keep a journal. Together they were to keep track of the family dinners (see appendix for menu ideas). Mim promised to either write down everything she ate away from home or tell her mom, who agreed to keep the record for her. Finally, I started Mim on the three supplements found in Dr. Erika's Essential Elements for teens (L-carnitine, coenzyme Q_{10}, and omega-3).

I saw Mim again in one month. She looked a little better and was even a little more tolerant of her family. Together we reviewed her journal.

It looked disastrous.

There were no family dinners. Mim didn't eat with her family. Either she took a plate of food to her room if she was around and liked what her mother had prepared, or she went out with her friends for fast food. Soda was a staple, and Diet Coke her favorite.

Since she stopped the birth control pills, she hadn't had a period. She wasn't concerned, she just felt bloated. Her weight hadn't changed yet.

My advice after the second visit was the following:

1. Start natural progesterone (200 milligrams in transdermal cream form) every evening until she gets her period.
2. Continue the supplements.
3. Continue keeping a journal.
4. Decrease the amount of soda by one serving a day.
5. Eat dinner at home with the family two nights a week.
6. When going out with friends, opt for salads or grilled foods instead of fried ones. Use oil and wine vinegar for dressing.
7. Increase water intake to five to eight glasses a day.

Mim followed my advice. When I saw her again a month later, she had lost two pounds and gotten her period twice, two weeks apart. At first she was a little annoyed with the frequency of the period, but when she realized she was feeling better and was reassured that her body was only rebalancing itself, she became okay with the trade-off—more frequent periods for better moods and less bloating.

Other things were changing in Mim's life as well. She started to join the family for dinner. At first it was only once a week, but it shortly became three or four times. She did cut down on the soda, and while she didn't stop going out with her friends, she started eating salads at both the pizza parlor and McDonald's. She also increased her water intake dramatically.

Over the following three years Mim suffered a few setbacks.

At times increasing levels of stress would cause her to start eating junk food and soda again. Initially I would find out from her mother about it, but in time Mim came to tell me about her so-called relapses on her own.

To help her get back on track, we went back to record-keeping, and over a period of a week or two she decreased the amount of soda and junk food. As Mim became aware of how much better she felt when she followed my advice, the setbacks became more infrequent.

Overall, Mim lost twenty pounds and kept them off. She also went off medication for her psychological problems and started doing better in school.

In time she changed peer groups and became friends with a more conventional group of teens.

She started working out, and by the age of seventeen she had a steady boyfriend and was looking at colleges with good teaching programs. She wanted to become a middle school teacher to help teens like herself negotiate the tough years without the help of medications or behavioral problem labels.

Mim was remarkably successful because she was motivated, she had a great family support system, and her mother was able to identify the root cause of her problems. Had her mother not realized the hormone connection between the start of her period and the beginning of Mim's problems, it would have been difficult for Mim to weather the adolescent storm so well.

Sometimes, though, the support system that is so critical is missing, and that is when teens rebel and the rebellion just doesn't stop.

Carmen was sixteen when I met her. Her mother brought her to me to help her lose weight.

Carmen came from a wealthy family. Her parents were financially successful, and she never lacked for material things. For her birthday she received a BMW, and she had her own credit card and access to unlimited funds. All that was expected of her was not to embarrass her family, and being overweight was considered unacceptable. Her mother was beautiful and thin, and her father was perfectly trim and fit. They both worked out with a professional trainer.

Carmen was overweight. She was on the track and lacrosse teams, she took piano lessons, and she was a skier and tennis player. The first time we met Carmen told me she was sure I couldn't help her. She had been to nutritionists, endocrinologists, and diet doctors. All attempts to help her had failed.

Carmen had irregular periods. She was sexually active, and her gynecologist had placed her on birth control pills to both regulate her period and prevent undesired pregnancy. Her weight increased more rapidly after she went on the birth control pills.

As a first step in my therapy, I asked Carmen to go off the birth control pills and keep a journal of her eating habits for a month. For birth control and prevention of sexually transmitted diseases, I recommended condoms.

While she agreed to go off the pills, she told me she'd never keep a journal. Her mother agreed with Carmen. I was asking far too much. They didn't have the time to comply with my request. Their lives were too busy to take the time to write things down for me.

They agreed to give me a month off the birth control pills, and if that approach seemed to help Carmen's weight problem, they might consider doing more with me. If not, they would move on to the next expert or therapy.

Under the circumstances, I thought anything they agreed to do would be helpful. I asked both mother and daughter to tell me about the family diet and lifestyle and said I would write down these details for them.

Carmen's parents traveled a lot, and they seldom ate together as a family. If they were home at the same time, they usually had different schedules, so family dinners were not an option in Carmen's treatment plan. Carmen just grabbed something on her way out to some after-school activity. She ate lots of high-protein or high-sugar and -fat candy bars.

Carmen was raised by a nanny from the Dominican Republic who cooked lots of fried, high-fat, high-calorie foods. She told me she often ate leftovers from the nanny's meals because that was the only thing in the house.

The open bar at home was also something Carmen considered a source of nutrition. She saw her parents drinking every time they were home, so she drank as well.

I advised her to stop drinking and asked her mother if she saw any way the family could get involved and help Carmen. I assured her that setting better eating and drinking examples would be the most helpful treatment for Carmen. I was asking for a higher level of commitment from Carmen's parents to be an active support system and set a better example for their daughter.

Carmen's mother told me she couldn't commit to family dinners because her schedule was too busy. She did, however, suggest bringing in a cook who could make healthy meals for Carmen. Unfortunately, Carmen would most likely have to eat by herself before running out to her activities. I agreed it was better than nothing, but I also knew this was not the solution Carmen desperately needed.

Carmen did lose a little weight. She did try to follow my advice for a few weeks, and her mother did hire the healthy food cook.

Unfortunately, they were all looking for a quick fix that couldn't be found without the emotional commitment of a family support system. Money cannot buy commitment or an emotional support system.

Carmen stopped coming to me after a few months. She had made nice progress during her time with me. She did lose ten pounds, I placed her on a couple of months of natural progesterone and supplements, and she did start keeping a journal.

She became more aware of the ingredients in her diet that helped her lose weight and those that didn't. She also gained a little insight into her family structure and saw that she was lacking support there.

Preserving Your Relationship with Your Teen While Trying to Help

Maura was sixteen and thirty pounds overweight. Her mother was also seriously overweight, and her presence in my consultation room was overbearing. Maura's mother, Olla, was from eastern Europe and took copious notes.

Olla brought every book I've written to the consultation. She had marked the pages she found pertinent to her daughter's condition. She also brought in articles by various other hormone and nutrition experts. In all my years in practice, I had never met a more prepared patient. She had done her homework, and everything she said was correct. She understood the connection between hormones and weight gain. She knew how insulin, cortisol, estrogen, and progesterone interact.

She identified the times in Maura's cycle when Maura was

ovulating and connected those times to Maura's increase in symptoms: a rapid increase in weight, bloating, PMS, headaches, acne, and mood swings.

Listening to Olla, I felt she didn't need me to do anything more than write the prescription for the natural progesterone.

While Olla was expounding, I looked at Maura and suddenly understood that her mother's overzealous preparation was making an important contribution to Maura's problems. Maura was a project for her. Helping Maura was not the priority. Researching her problems was.

I don't mean to be harsh here. I have no doubt that Olla adored her daughter and believed she was helping. Unfortunately, her daughter felt lost, and what she needed most was a mother, not another expert on her problems. They had hired me to fill that need.

I couldn't say that to Olla on their first visit.

I asked Maura if she wanted to see me alone or with Olla at the next visit. When I received a resounding "I would like to see you alone," I seized the opportunity.

When we met the next time, we spoke about her mother. Maura told me her mother made her crazy with her weight problem. While she agreed she had a problem, she didn't understand why her mother was focusing so much on it.

She clearly was embarrassed, if not mortified, by the weight problem, but her mother's obsession with it upset Maura and distanced her from her mother and made her avoid solving the problem.

Maura preferred to talk to me about her level of energy, the pimples on her back, her irregular periods, and her school and social issues.

We spent six months speaking of everything but the weight problem. While we didn't speak of her weight, we did everything we could together to reduce her weight and improve her overall condition.

Maura found the solution in the following directions I gave her:

1. Take natural progesterone for three cycles.
2. Take supplements for six months.
3. Eat family dinners together (see appendix for menus).
4. Cut out soda and increase water intake.
5. Spend quality time with people she feels comfortable with and who are kind, supportive, and noncritical or judgmental of her.

Maura lost weight without speaking of it while all her other complaints vanished as well. Her pimples disappeared, her periods became more regular, her moods stabilized, and her energy level soared.

After my fourth session with Maura, I asked her if I could meet with her mother alone. Maura agreed but asked me not to give her mother too many details of our conversations together.

Olla came to our meeting armed with a tape recorder and a notebook. She didn't want to miss a word. I must admit that her excitement with the project she had turned her daughter into was infectious.

We spoke for more than an hour. Olla wanted to help but didn't see that she was more of a stumbling block than a helper. I told her that the best way she could help her daughter was to be her mother, not her doctor.

I then brought up her own weight problems. Grateful that I

noticed and was willing to talk about it, Olla told me she had had weight problems since her midthirties (she was forty-six when I first met her). Just like her daughter (keep in mind the importance of genetics), she suffered from hormone imbalances, and her focus on her daughter's weight was a distraction from focusing on her own issues.

Olla also wanted my help. We worked on her hormone problems, getting her balanced by placing her on a different combination of natural hormones that included natural progesterone as well as a form of estrogen called estradiol. We worked together on a family diet that would benefit the entire family.

Olla and her husband were ahead of the curve. They knew how important it was to connect with the children. They had raised their children with nightly family dinners. At the dinner table they talked about their day and did not focus on the food.

They had the foundation for great support for the children and were committed to helping. Olla was just lacking the right tools.

Coming from eastern Europe, Olla was very traditional in the types of foods she fed her family. Their meals had high starch content and included lots of bread, polenta, pasta, and potatoes. They ate large portions with high quantities of animal fat and meats. She fried most meats in lots of butter and oil.

Olla more than willingly kept a food journal for me. Once I knew the weak points in their diet, I was able to guide her to implement much-needed changes.

Olla and her family became one of the model families that led me to the family menus you find in the appendix. Olla not only helped Maura, she helped herself, her husband, and her two other children, younger boys who were entering their teen age at the time we were working together.

The stories in this chapter serve to show the importance of integrating all parts of your teen's life to give her the best support to weather teen rebellion, weight management, and hormone balance. With the increased awareness we have gained, I know you will find the threat of teen rebellion less ominous and more of a challenge you now know you can and will successfully meet.

9

Sex, Drugs, and Rock and Roll

On January 19, 2004, Ellen Waterston, the author of *Then There Was No Mountain: The Parallel Odyssey of a Mother and Daughter Through Addiction*, appeared on *Good Morning, America*. She spoke of her personal struggle as a mother in the world of drug-addicted children.

Having decided to leave her drug-addict husband with her three small children (ages ten, eight, and five) to save them from their father's influence, Waterston believed she could protect her children by keeping them busy and avoiding the topic of drugs and addiction. She moved from the family farm she had shared with her husband in Oregon with the goal of creating a world where her husband's drug problems didn't exist. Through denial and convoluted thinking that prevented her from facing the truth that her husband was a drug addict, she became involved in deceptive and dishonest relationships with herself and the world around her. Handicapped by her own issues, she was unable to provide the foundation her children needed to protect themselves from the underworld of drugs.

Unfortunately for both her and the children, peer pressure prevailed: her middle child and youngest child succumbed to drug addiction. In the book, Waterston honestly admits to her own addiction to guilt, control, and victimization (anything we use as a crutch to deny the truth about ourselves and avoid taking responsibility for our lives is an addiction) and makes a rarely seen connection between her personal problems as a parent and the resulting drug problems her children developed.

Waterston addresses not only the recovery process her daughter had to go through but also the changes she as a parent had to make to truly help her daughter. "Parenting is not a popularity contest," Waterston tells her readers.

She is right, and this statement is by far the single most important lesson a parent must learn when making a realistic commitment to raising an emotionally intact human being. Honesty is a basic requirement, and constant, truthful evaluation of yourself, your teen, and your relationship is crucial to success.

Lee was sixteen when her mother brought her to see me. She had been in rehab three times since age fourteen. She was addicted to marijuana and alcohol and on occasion took prescription painkillers and diet pills. She had a weight problem, and her hormones were out of balance (her periods were irregular and she had acne and PMS). Lee's mother brought her to me for the sole purpose of balancing her hormones.

Growing up, Lee had been a model child. She came from a well-educated New England family. Her father was a highly regarded college professor, her mother was an adjunct, and the family lived on campus. Lee was the third of four children. Lee's parents groomed their children to follow in their footsteps and become academics. They were involved with numerous activities, including sports, dance, and acting. Dinner was a nightly requirement that Lee and her brothers often felt they needed a written excuse to miss. The family was very formal. Children were expected to dress for dinner. No caps or jeans were allowed.

Lee's parents used dinner as a forum to educate their children and establish their point of view and expectations. The children's duties were clear and simple to the parents: they had to perform well in school and follow the parents' rules without question. The family was not a democracy.

Lee fit into the family mold until she turned thirteen. That year she started menstruating, and everything about her changed. She gained weight, she developed a mild but persistent case of acne, and her periods and moods became unpredictable.

The family ignored the changes in Lee. They had two older boys, and they too had changed when they entered adolescence. The boys' voices changed, and they had become withdrawn and even less communicative than they had been as children. Lee's parents weren't concerned—they were boys, after all, and their personalities were not a family issue. As long as they performed well in school, everything was all right.

Unlike her brothers, Lee tried to speak with her mother about her unhappiness with her body and looks. When her mother casually dismissed Lee's concerns by telling her looks weren't important, Lee stopped sharing her feelings with her.

At school Lee had been an excellent student until she started to menstruate and her world came crashing down on her. With the change in moods and her weight gain, she was unable to stay focused on schoolwork, and her thinking became cloudy.

She was starting to have trouble in math, and out of embarrassment and fear she decided not to tell her parents. Up to the time she started her period, her girlfriends were a group of top-performing students. When Lee started to show signs of trouble, she became estranged from her old friends.

Feeling that she didn't belong with the same group any longer, Lee moved toward a different group of girls. The new group weren't good students or popular, like the first group—they were on the fringe.

In particular she was drawn to a girl who also had a weight problem but seemed to always be in a good mood and willing to listen and offer advice. Disappointed with herself and her mother's reaction, Lee was desperately looking for an ear and a shoulder at this point.

The girl was the answer to Lee's prayers. In a few weeks they became fast friends, and soon after the girl took her into her confidence. The girl's mother had taken her to a diet doctor, who had given her diet pills. The girl believed that they worked and that they also helped her focus better in school.

Lee borrowed some pills from her new friend. She didn't lose any weight, but she enjoyed the rush and the high energy level she had for hours after taking a pill. Lee began to emulate her new best friend's habits.

It took no time for Lee to start drinking and smoking marijuana with her new girlfriend. She found the girl's group more accepting than her former friends or her own family.

When Lee complained about her family, her new friends listened and empathized. They offered her drugs and alcohol, and Lee took them even though she knew her family wouldn't approve. Strangely, the thrill seemed to come from doing exactly what she had been told not to do.

Lee was spending more time with her new friends and less time at school or at home. She started missing dinner. She made up stories and became entangled in a web of lies.

At first her mother believed her tales of extra schoolwork. Soon, however, her behavior became more suspect. She was always late, her personality changed, and she developed a bad temper. She became unreliable and disinterested in her physical appearance. Her body hygiene deteriorated as well.

Lee was in trouble in school and at home, and the only place she felt secure was with her friends and their drugs.

One phone call from school to her parents brought out the truth. Both parents and school officials agreed that Lee had a serious drug problem.

Without even speaking with Lee, her parents picked her up from school and took her to a rehab program in Connecticut. She was fourteen. By the time Lee turned sixteen, she had been in three different rehab programs.

She was trouble-free in rehab, but as soon as she went home she fell off the wagon.

Medication, therapy, and clinical supervision didn't seem to be able to keep Lee from her drugs.

Her family was disgusted at Lee's behavior, and when I first saw her, her mother told me her father was considering disowning Lee.

I felt sorry for Lee. She was a pretty girl with very sad eyes without sparkle. She looked more like fifty than sixteen. Being the hormone expert on the case, I felt restricted in what I could offer. Her mother clearly only wanted to have her daughter's hormones balanced and help her lose some weight if possible.

I did place Lee on natural progesterone for two months and

added the customary supplements (L-carnitine, coenzyme Q-10, and omega-3). Before Lee and her mother left, I also added a piece of advice. I told Lee's mother that I strongly believed her daughter desperately needed a mother who accepted her as a person and listened to her needs.

Setting rules is an integral part of parenting when the kids are small and need continuous guidance and direction. As children get older, things change; support and acceptance for a teen's individual needs must be combined with a loosening of the parental rules to help the teen successfully negotiate adolescence.

Support, guidance, and a parent who listens and confronts the truth at all times without fear is the only hope a teen has.

Lee's mother needed to talk to Lee and acknowledge her daughter's feelings even if her needs were not what the mother wanted them to be. I suggested that she provide some warmth and comfort to her daughter. I also suggested that Lee didn't have to fit into the family mold to be okay. Accepting Lee and encouraging her to be less self-destructive was going to prove more helpful than drug-rehab programs.

I also stressed with Lee's mother that the weight problem was of enormous concern to Lee, and discounting it had sent her directly into the arms of the drug user and occasional dealer friend.

Lee's mother heard me.

The last time I saw Lee was three years later. She had been drug-free since we began working together, and she had lost the weight she referred to as "baby weight." Lee was a freshman at Yale and wanted to become an actress. While her relationship with her father hadn't improved much, Lee and her mother had become very close.

What You the Parent Want to Know
Versus What You Should Know

Jill was sixteen when she came for a physical examination accompanied by her mother. She was healthy and pretty, but also a little overweight and wearing loose-fitting sweats. At first glance, I thought something wasn't right with Jill. Her weight seemed oddly distributed on her body. She looked pregnant to me.

Jill's mother had worked with me at the hospital for years. She was a highly regarded and competent nurse. Every physician wanted her to care for his/her patients. I pushed the thought of Jill being pregnant out of my mind.

During the examination it became apparent that I wasn't wrong. Jill had a little belly and, I discovered on palpation, a pregnant uterus. Not wanting to believe my own eyes and hands, I ran into the laboratory with Jill's urine specimen and performed a quick pregnancy test. It was positive.

I asked Jill when she had had her last period. Casually she said she didn't keep exact track, but she thought sometime within the last month. I told her I had good reason to believe she was pregnant. She looked surprised and said she wasn't. Her periods had been irregular, but she denied having unprotected sex. The issue of sex was academic, and I told her we had to address the situation with her mother.

Jill shrugged her shoulders in what I chose to read as approval.

When I told Jill's mother that her daughter was pregnant, she couldn't believe it. She was truly shocked.

I must admit I was more shocked than both my patient and her mother. I couldn't understand how this mother, who was a nurse and lived in the same house with her daughter, had failed to notice the daughter's developing pregnancy.

Jill and her mother would go through traumatic years together. The pregnancy was only the beginning of years of trouble, drug addiction, and alcoholism. As the years unfolded, Jill's mother told me that she didn't want to know that her daughter was troubled, so she convinced herself everything was all right. In time, when she couldn't deny Jill's problems any longer, she could see them but was afraid of Jill's reaction to confrontation, so she chose not to ask.

Jill became more troubled with every passing month, and I followed them for only a short while. The care they needed involved therapy, rehabilitation centers, and special schools.

Jill's story is one that I bring to you from years ago, when I was practicing internal medicine. But it is just as pertinent today, if not more so.

Parents must know as much as possible about the lives of their teenagers. Giving teens privacy cannot mean letting them go through their hardest years without guidance and supervision.

It is often easier to close our eyes than to deal with an unexpected or unwanted reality. However, if we don't address the problem the moment we see it, it will only escalate and the teen will become more troubled.

The lesson I learned from my experience with Jill and her mother was threefold.

1. Good parenting is about communication and paying attention.
2. Good parenting is about never being afraid of your child.

3. Good parenting translates into healthy, well-adjusted teens.

How to Set Up a Dialogue with Your Teen

The key to setting up a dialogue with your teen is to be relentless.

Corey was fourteen when she told her mother to stop butting into her life. Corey was not doing well in school, and her mother wasn't happy with her friends and new college-age boyfriend.

I was seeing Corey because she was overweight and her periods were irregular. I knew from the first visit that getting through to Corey was going to be no small feat. She sat sullenly in the chair facing me with downcast eyes. Regardless of what I said, Corey grunted and her mother acted as if there was nothing wrong with Corey's behavior.

Before I could do my job, I had to get through to Corey. The only way I could get through to her was to help her mother get through to her first. I asked Corey's mother to call me.

She was so happy that I wanted to talk about her daughter. She found it difficult to engage her other doctors in conversation about Corey. Her pediatrician had said that all teens were the same and that in time Corey would either come around or not. Not very reassuring for Corey's mother. My advice was simple.

- Be relentless. Never give up. "If your daughter won't talk to you, talk to her. And keep talking until she starts responding, even if it takes a long time."
- Don't be intrusive or aggressive. While respecting her privacy, don't leave her unattended or unsupervised.
- Give her room, but keep coming back to her and ask how she is doing.

- If you see she isn't doing well, make your observations known.
- Don't be judgmental—just be honest and kind. ("Kind doesn't mean dishonest—it means truthful without being hurtful.)
- Be compassionate and accepting of the differences between you and your daughter, but always stress kindness and honesty as universal requirements.

Corey and her mother connected after a few months. Corey took natural progesterone for three cycles, and her family started eating the foods I recommend in the appendix. Corey joined a gym with her mom and after another six months stopped seeing the boyfriend.

How to Gain Your Teen's Trust

The only way to gain another person's trust is by being honest and consistent.

Your teen may look and act differently than adults do, but just like every other human, she will react positively to honesty and consistency.

Donna Mae was thirteen and had been in and out of foster homes too many times to count. She was a troubled teen I was seeing for nutritional counseling and hormone balance at a clinic I was working at.

Donna Mae was not an unusual case. Her life was too hard for her age. No child should have to go through such trauma. Unfortunately, she is one of too many. She never followed my advice, and I often felt defeated when leaving the clinic.

About six months into our work together, Donna Mae hadn't

lost one ounce. She kept forgetting to take her progesterone. She became more bloated and moody. I saw her around Christmas, when she told me she was being sent to live with a new family. She wasn't sure it was going to work, but she was hopeful. I wished her well and said a little prayer for her on my way out of the clinic.

The next time I saw Donna Mae was in June of the following year. She had lost ten pounds, looked positively radiant, and was coming to thank me for my help. She also wanted to introduce me to her new mother. I was so happy to see her and wanted to know what had happened to produce such miraculous improvement in her. She was now fourteen and a half, and by all rights she should have been in the midst of massive turmoil.

Donna Mae had found the right family. Her new parents were kind and decent and showed interest in her. Her new mother honestly told me that she had never dealt with a teen before but wanted to help and needed all the direction I could offer. She had stood by Donna Mae and reinforced her in all the activities that helped her while gently dissuading her from destructive actions. Donna Mae was following the advice I had given her a year earlier. Unfortunately, the first time I saw Donna Mae her life has been too chaotic and unsettled for her to follow my advice. Now, in the proper nurturing environment, she was taking progesterone and supplements, cooking dinner with her new mom, and even working out three times a week.

There was no further advice for me to give. They certainly were in a position to give advice to the rest of us.

Reality and Adequate Protection

Sybil has been one of my patients for many years. She came to ask me for help with her daughter's contraception. Sybil's gynecologist had offered to start the sexually active sixteen-year-old on birth control pills, but Sybil wasn't comfortable with that and asked for my help in the hope that I could place her daughter on natural hormones and provide contraception for her.

I couldn't. Unlike synthetic birth control pills, which override the body's natural hormonal cycle, natural hormones support the natural cycle and thus cannot be used for contraception.

My advice, based on the reality that Sybil's daughter was sexually active, was that the girl needed to use condoms and Sybil had to teach her daughter to be careful and selective about her sexuality.

Condoms are the best all-around protection we have for our sexually active teens. Condoms protect from most sexually transmitted diseases, and they also prevent pregnancy if properly used. They are not the solution to promiscuity and lack of self-esteem.

One of the significant parts of protection is education. Teaching your teen to have high self-esteem is the key. Being realistic in her expectations and needs is crucial to obtaining true protection.

Sexually Transmitted Diseases and AIDS—Not Your Teen

No book on teens can be complete without at least a section on sexually transmitted diseases and HIV.

I have yet to meet a parent who believes there is even the remotest of possibilities her daughter could be at risk for STDs or HIV. I wish I could feel as confident as all the parents I meet. I always wonder, whose children get these dreadful diseases?

Working in offices, clinics, and hospitals over the past thirty years, I have seen more than my share of teens with sexually transmitted diseases and AIDS. They weren't all underprivileged or abandoned.

One of my first cases of AIDS was an eighteen-year-old college student. She came to see me with a persistent dry cough during a school break. She had been tired for months, and her mother kept blaming the college lifestyle for her daughter's plight. We took a chest X-ray to see why she had the cough. It showed pneumocystis pneumonia, which is a type of pneumonia typical of AIDS.

The diagnosis was devastating not only to the patient but to her whole family and the clinical staff who were taking care of her. We all felt betrayed. She was a beautiful, smart, and vivacious young woman we had all known since her childhood. It just could not be.

She had had a few sex partners but was not promiscuous. One evening after a big party at college she went home with a guy she met. It was the first time for her, and they had sex without a condom. Two months later she started complaining of being tired all the time. It was quick, but unfortunately not unusual. Six months later I had the misfortune of having to bring the family the deadly news.

Her parents never believed their daughter was sexually active, let alone that she could have AIDS. How could this have happened to their daughter?

I cannot stress the importance of educating our teens about sexually transmitted diseases and instilling into them the reality of the danger in every casual sexual encounter.

STDs and AIDS do happen, and they happen to teens more than any other age group. Your teen doesn't have to be an IV drug user or be sexually promiscuous. Every time she has unprotected sex she is at risk!

Drugs

We live in a drug- and alcohol-infested culture. Our teen's role models are celebrities who are in and out of rehab centers, musicians and rich kids seen with a glass of alcohol in hand in every picture in the most popular magazines. All our culture encourages our teens to do is have fun, and that translates into drugs, alcohol, and sex. Every reality show they watch involves drinking and partying.

There is no prize or reward placed on maintaining a drug- and alcohol-free life. The only teens who don't drink or do drugs seem to be the ones who have gone through rehab or are considered geeks.

Maybe this is an exaggeration of the situation, but I mention it because I must make a very important point.

It seems unreasonable and even delusional to believe your teen will not be exposed to drugs and alcohol, that she will not try them, or, worst of all, that she might not get seriously entangled in them.

Sylvia was eighteen when her mother brought her to me to help balance her hormones. She had gained ten pounds during her first semester at college, her periods were irregular, and she had acne. Before leaving for college, Sylvia had no problems. She had been a good student, even if academic success came at the expense of not being popular in school. When she went off to college, something changed. After the first few weeks of homesickness and continuous phone calls to her mother, Sylvia underwent a remarkable change. She became close friends with her roommate, a girl from an inner-city fast crowd. Sylvia suddenly loved everything about college, especially her roommate.

She stopped calling her mother. When her mom was able to

catch up with her on the phone, Sylvia was always in a rush but reassured her mother that everything was going great and she was extremely happy in school. Relieved, her mother believed everything Sylvia said.

When Sylvia returned home for Thanksgiving, her mother was stunned. Her daughter had purple hair streaks and multiple piercings, she had gained weight, and her face was covered with acne.

My first question to Sylvia was about drugs and alcohol. She vociferously denied being involved in them. Her mother was offended and told me she had no doubt that her daughter would never get involved in that type of behavior.

Although I tried to help Sylvia by giving her natural hormones and recommending ways to improve her college diet, she didn't improve much.

At Christmas, Sylvia's mother came to see me, crying. Sylvia was having problems in school, and when confronted by her mother, she finally confessed she was drinking every day and smoking marijuana as well.

Her mother kept her home the following semester, and with counseling and honest family support, she helped Sylvia disengage from the friends she had made at college and find her balance back with her family. She switched schools and had no further problems.

The point of Sylvia's story is simple but crucial to saving our teens from the dangers of drugs and alcohol.

- *All* our teens *are* exposed to drugs and alcohol. Unless you are planning on keeping them in a protective bubble, you cannot avoid this reality of teen life in the United States in 2004.

- Being honest and confronting your teen when you observe incongruous, strange changes in her personality and physical presence are key.

- It isn't easier to deny what you see. It will not go away. So face the truth as soon as you see a change and do not let go of it. You are the parent, and your teen desperately needs your guidance. If you are wrong, the worst that can happen is that your teen will get angry with you. If you are right, you may have stopped the domino effect from robbing your child of her health and innocence.

- Be there for your teen. Ask questions and deal with the truth. You'll save her life.

- You must teach your teen to be safe within herself. That means being honest with herself and you! Safety comes from the inside. Safe behavior is always connected to being aware, clear-headed, and honest.

- Build your teen's self-esteem. Teens who feel good about themselves and have support and a solid foundation don't get into bad trouble. Chances are, they will all experiment, but if their self-esteem is high, they will not hurt themselves.

Dating

Our adolescents travel in packs. They don't date in the classic way that we, their parents, used to do. This cultural difference provides a certain level of comfort and is probably evolutionary. Girls and boys are friends, and the pressure of having a date on Friday or Saturday night is no longer a source of competition.

Weight, looks, and dress, however, are important determinants of the group your teen belongs to. Everyone strives to be part of the "in" group. Popularity is defined by who your friends are.

Betsy was fifteen when her mother brought her to me. She had been gaining weight progressively over two years in spite of her parents' continuous and committed efforts. The moment Betsy started to show signs of weight gain, her parents completely revamped their eating habits and cleaned the junk food out of the cupboards. Her mother joined a gym with Betsy and made sure the two worked out religiously twice a week. All to no avail.

Betsy got her period at thirteen and until then had been thin. She belonged to the most popular group of girls in her middle school class and was on every sports team. The day she got her period everything changed. Betsy's mood changed, and her bright disposition and constant smile vanished.

She started to gain weight, and her friends stopped inviting her to go out with them. The more she was ostracized by her group, the more junk she ate, and the more depressed and overweight she became.

By the time I saw her for her irregular periods, acne, and weight gain, Betsy was far from thin or friendly. Her gaze was fixed on the floor, and her clothes, all oversized, were a telltale sign of her self-confidence problem.

Betsy was becoming less confident and more embarrassed by her weight every day. Instead of trying to lose the weight and work to succeed, she had given up and felt helpless. She didn't even want to talk about the weight problem.

I worked with Betsy for almost a year. Initially all I addressed was her hormone issue. We worked with natural progesterone for a few months to get her period in better balance. Her acne started to resolve, and her moods improved.

We added the usual supplements (L-carnitine, coenzyme Q_{10}, and omega-3). Betsy felt better. Her energy levels improved, and by the second month we were talking about school and her family.

It still took another two months before she spoke to me about her weight and her friends. She was so pained and sad about the impact of her weight on her relationships with other girls and boys and on her status in her peer group that she didn't know what to do.

In time I found myself working more on helping Betsy develop her self-esteem than on watching her diet. I reassured her about herself and her future success at keeping her weight within normal range for her.

The better she felt about the prospect that she would lose weight and eventually be accepted by the popular girls, the more she became involved in changing her eating habits for the better and increasing her exercise regimen. Once she had hope, she aimed for success.

By the end of the year Betsy had lost ten pounds. She had significantly improved her self-esteem, and her confidence started to soar. She went away with friends skiing, and she became more popular. She was still pudgy, but she didn't feel unsightly, and she didn't sabotage her own efforts to keep her weight down. She became comfortable and satisfied with Betsy.

The growing problem with weight gain and the social pressures associated with being thin make a deadly combination for the average girl. Not everyone has the genetic material that will keep her thin throughout her adolescent years. Most girls will gain weight before they enter puberty. Remember, we must have a significant amount of body fat to get our periods! It's Mother Nature's mandate! We can't change that.

Depression and loss of self-confidence brought on by the social pressures of staying thin only make the transition to adulthood more difficult. Failure comes from a combination of feeling terrible about the natural weight gain that comes with the onset of puberty and the hormone changes that bring on the period and the inability to maintain a healthy diet in a society where our teens are surrounded by junk food.

Just as we saw with Betsy, there is hope.

- Keep encouraging your daughter. Do not obsess about weight and social status issues.
- By example, keep healthy foods in your house and throw out the junk.
- If you don't like her friends, tell her. Do it kindly and explain why you don't like them.
- Accept your daughter's decision about her friends and stand by when you are proven right to give her support, not to rub salt in her wounds.
- Give her hope! She will succeed if you believe she will.

10

Fathers and Daughters

Cornelia was fourteen when her father noted at the dinner table, in front of family and friends, that she had put on weight and her skin looked bad.

Cornelia was a lovely teen girl I had been treating for acne and weight gain that started around the time she began menstruating. With the help of natural progesterone and a good dermatologist, we had been able to reduce her acne and were now working to help her lose the weight.

Cornelia and her mother had been working very diligently, following the menus in the appendix of this book and increasing Cornelia's physical activity. The results were starting to show, and we all agreed that Cornelia was well on her way to being an overall happier teen. She was doing well in school, and her self-esteem was at an all-time high after six intensive months of working together.

When she told me about her father's insensitive remark, I was taken aback but unfortunately not surprised.

How Do Fathers Deal with the Changes in "Daddy's Little Girl"?

Cornelia's story is more common than any of us would like it to be. Somehow, in their attempt to be good fathers, many men miss the mark on the sensitivity factor.

When I started telling my friends and colleagues I was writing a book on teens and the increasing problem with weight they are experiencing, every mother and teen girl, without exception, asked me to include a section on fathers. The stories came pouring in. And they all contained the same fears and disappointments with father–teen daughter relationships.

Sasha was seventeen and came from a highly educated, high-achieving family. Both her parents were professionals, and she was their only child. Success in school was expected of Sasha. She was sent to the best private school and her performance in school was closely watched. Sasha was very close to her mother—the two represented a unit of love and support for each other.

Sasha came to see me because she was putting on weight, her periods were irregular, and her skin was developing acne. Before seeing me, Sasha's mother had taken her to the pediatrician and the endocrinologist. A diagnosis of possible insulin-resistance was made. The doctors had performed many blood tests, and after the results showed increased levels of testosterone, Sasha was sent off with the unsatisfactory recommendation, "We'll see how you are in six months."

Sasha's mother took action. They went to a university-based teen weight reduction clinic. Sasha felt out of place. The other girls attending the clinic were obese, while Sasha needed to lose only fifteen to twenty pounds.

Sasha's mother realized that her daughter needed overall balancing, including hormones, supplements, diet, exercise, and lifestyle adjustment, instead of the unilateral focus of the weight reduction clinic or the wait-and-see physician recommendation. She brought her daughter to me.

Sasha responded well to my advice. I worked with her to learn as much about her whole life as possible and then started giving her guidance to help her integrate all the pieces. She took natural progesterone for her irregular periods and started on the supplements to help increase her energy. Within a month Sasha got her period, her face started to clear up, and her energy level improved.

We could now address her diet. Increasing her protein and complex carbohydrate intake, while eliminating some of the junk food, further improved the situation. Her physical activity level was not very high, so we made little changes there as well.

She lived in an apartment building on a high floor. We decided, no more elevators. After another two months Sasha was looking better and feeling even better than she looked. Her eyes had their shine back, and her general outlook had improved.

Her weight was starting to come off while her self-image and hormone balance were getting better as well.

A wonderful success story? Not quite.

On a routine follow-up visit ten weeks later, Sasha looked withdrawn and distanced. When I asked her what was wrong, she meekly told me she knew she would always have a weight problem. I was baffled. There was no reason for her to have become so negative so suddenly. I probed a little deeper.

The answer, unfortunately, did not come as a surprise to me.

Sasha told me that her father had told her she was fat. And not only once but numerous times. When she was trying on a more revealing, or what she called "cute," outfit, he ridiculed her and made rude, insensitive comments. Sasha told me that was the way her family functioned. Her father constantly grumbled about her mother's and Sasha's imperfections. He was condescending and critical about everything Sasha felt was important. He complained about her looks, her performance in school, her friends, her relationship with her mother, everything.

I wanted to know if Sasha remembered a good time with her father. She thought for a while, and then, unsure of herself, she said, "Maybe when I was much younger."

Sasha's story is more common than you would think.

Fathers and daughters are lost in the transition of the daughter from "little princess" to adolescent female. I find it uncomfortably rare to find a supportive father who doesn't suddenly either withdraw from the budding woman or begin a frontal attack on her, just because she no longer fits the image of his little girl.

I want to believe fathers really want to help their daughters grow up into self-assured, comfortable young women. I want to believe it is lack of advice and direction from professionals or attention from all of us that has caused the situation to deteriorate this far.

I would like to never see another teenage girl come into my office crying because her father told her she is fat, or another mother telling me she wants to kill her husband because all he does is belittle her and her daughter on a regular basis.

As a physician and a mother of two girls, I have personally experienced the nefarious effects of negative male comments and behavior on both my daughters and me.

The negative experiences haven't stopped me from maintaining my positive attitude. I hold out hope for fathers and am committed to providing guidance and help to the fathers and daughters lost in the storm of adolescence.

Fathers, your daughter needs you and you cannot afford to lose your little girl now. Take my advice: I assure you that your daughter and her mother will thank you. The results will amaze you, and your relationship with women will improve overnight!

Following my advice will help your daughter develop a better self-image and more confidence and will prepare her for good and successful relationships with boys. Isn't that what you really want and need to give her?

- Think before you speak. Your daughter is sensitive, and everything you say she reacts to on an emotional level. When you think you are being honest and supportive, you may be destructive and hurtful.
- Understand that teenage girls are extremely self-conscious about their appearance and body image. Any references to appearance or body image should be positive and reassuring. If you don't have anything positive to say, don't say anything at all. Lying is not an option. Let your daughter start the conversation about sensitive issues. If she doesn't, wait. Bring up her strong points. Find her strong points.
- Discuss concerns about your daughter with her mother. Even when the relationship between mother and daughter is at its most difficult, chances are that her mother has a little more insight into how your daughter is feeling. Working together will benefit your daughter, and that is the goal.

- The relationship between you and your daughter will shape the relationships she has with other males. If you are not supportive or loving toward your daughter, she will seek support and love in shallow, short-term relationships that place her at risk.

- Do not withdraw when your daughter becomes a teen. Don't be scared of the physical changes in her—she is still your girl. The time she needs you the most is when she starts becoming a woman. Gently reassure her about her appearance and encourage her to feel good about herself. Your support and emotional presence will accomplish more than years in therapy.

- Appearing scared or uninterested pushes the insecurity button in your daughter. She is the same person you loved to play with before she started to look like a woman. Don't make her feel awkward because her body has changed. If you are supportive, encouraging, and kind, she will not come home with blue hair and multiple piercings.

- Hear and listen to your daughter. She is no longer a baby, and although she still desperately needs your approval, she knows there are other ways to look at life than your way, no matter how successful you are. She doesn't always have to be wrong. You don't always have to be right.

- Spend time speaking with your daughter. Listen to her talk about her interests, boys, shopping, other girls, anything she wants to talk about. Every encounter with her is a teaching opportunity for you. Consider yourself lucky if she shares her life with you.

- Notice your daughter as a person in her own right, not as

an extension of her mother or you. Learn to see her as an individual. Treat her with respect.

- Accept your daughter.
- Don't push too hard, or you'll lose her.
- Acknowledge and reinforce your daughter's achievements and encourage her potential.
- If you are uncomfortable with a particular topic, say so to your daughter rather than avoid or deny its existence.
- Give her hope for her future.

Divorced Fathers

I raised my daughters alone. The choice to get divorced was mine. I tried being a superwoman and a wife but found out after a couple of tries that being a wife was not my forte.

At that time in my life I was very career-oriented. That was my personal impediment to married life and raising children with a husband.

I was raised in a conventional eastern European family and believed it was important that my daughters and I stay connected to their fathers. They were both professionals and committed to their daughters in principle. They generally showed up for their biweekly visits, took the girls on vacations, and came to school plays, games, and parents' evenings. Over the years we even had holidays together. My friends and patients marveled at my ability to maintain good relationships with my daughters' fathers. On occasion I did too.

The inevitable transition from little girls to teenagers and adult women occurred. I am sad to tell you that the relationships with their fathers became more and more tenuous with the passing years. As the girls grew up, I slowly removed myself from the relationship between my daughters and their fathers. I thought that in time the fathers would have their own independent relationships with the girls. I stopped making sure they called each other, and I stopped covering up for the fathers' insensitivities and occasional inconsistencies. I got remarried.

Once I was out of the picture and the girls and their fathers were left to their own resources, things started to fall apart. As you might imagine, I did not raise wallflowers. My daughters are outspoken, honest, and maybe a tad intolerant of inconsiderate or irresponsible behavior.

My older daughter's father was unable to accept her as an individual in her own right. In time he distanced himself from her life, and as of this writing he no longer participates in the joy of having her as a daughter. He missed her law school graduation, and they have no contact even though they live less than thirty miles apart.

My younger daughter, a college student and also a great woman in the making, has a cordial but almost indifferent relationship with her father. Years ago, when his older daughter graduated from college, I remember him lamenting over his distanced relationship with her. I said, "All you have is today, so make it better—it's all up to you!" At the time I also pointed out to him that he had another very young daughter and a little stepdaughter as well. He had two more chances to get it right. So far, unfortunately, he hasn't used that experience to improve his relationship with his younger daughter.

Although my personal experience with divorced men hasn't been the best, I still firmly believe that with help and true commitment, a divorced father can be a positive and crucial ingredient in his daughter's life and her transition from child to adult.

- Keep the lines of communication open with your daughter's mother. Your daughter needs you. Don't disappear from her life just because the relationship with her mother didn't work out.
- Be present in your daughter's life even if you are not physically there. Phone calls, e-mails, the written word, all count as connection. Do not miss any important times in her life—school plays, graduations, birthdays, games.
- Tell your daughter you care and back it up with actions. Lip service doesn't stand the test of time.
- Take responsibility for the success of your relationship with your daughter. Regardless of what you think, the outcome of your relationship with your daughter is 100 percent your own doing. Your daughter responds to you, so look at yourself and your behavior when evaluating the relationship.

Single Fathers

Loretta was raised by her father. Her mother left the family when Loretta was very young.

When I first saw Loretta, she was fourteen and twenty pounds overweight. She was referred to me by a family friend. Loretta was the mother in the family. She had a younger brother, and she took care of both her father's and brother's every need. When we started speaking of diets, Loretta quickly informed me that her father and brother ate only steak and potatoes and loved desserts. She could not change the menus to help herself lose weight because it would upset the men.

I next suggested that Loretta increase her physical activity.

There too I met with a negative reply. Loretta had no time because she had to go to school and then take care of the men.

Finally, exasperated, I asked Loretta to come to see me with her father at her next visit. She did. Her father was a lovely and very cooperative man.

Unfortunately for Loretta, her father had no idea how difficult her life was. He went to work in the morning and returned home at dinnertime. He didn't spend much time paying attention to the details of his well-organized life run by a fourteen-year-old.

When I pointed out to him that his life was orderly and under control at his daughter's expense, he was mortified.

Here was a father who wanted nothing more than to take good care of his children. I advised him to get a housekeeper and encourage Loretta to become a fourteen-year-old rather than the absent mother. He followed my advice and even started coming along to Loretta's appointments with me.

Loretta did very well. She lost the weight and became a regular teen.

Adolescence is a time of turmoil for both fathers and daughters. It is also an opportunity to reevaluate your relationship and program it for success. While the train to adulthood has left the station and your daughter is no longer a little girl, she needs you, and a solid relationship with you will give her a good foundation for success in relationships with men for the rest of her life. Don't miss out on it!

11

Boys Are Teens Too

Parents of both boys and girls consistently tell me that raising boys is easier than raising girls. They all agree on the reasons. Boys, I am told, are less moody, whiny, and emotional. Once a boy enters puberty, his focus turns to sports and his buddies. No matter what supermodel's picture he has hanging on his bedroom wall, a boy is not a victim of peer pressure or intimidation as often as a girl is.

Boys are also less communicative and more private, and many mothers quickly feel like outsiders in their sons' lives when they become teenagers. Apparently they expect this change and do not challenge it.

In our times of change, boys are not spared. They too are becoming overweight, and along with the growing weight problem we see changes in their hormone balance and social behavior.

Physical and Hormonal Changes That Bring the Boy into Adolescence

Before puberty, there is not much sexual difference between our children. We dress them differently and give them different toys to play with, but stripped of our social and cultural mores, little boys and girls are pretty similar in appearance.

Change starts with the onset of puberty. We now know in detail what happens at puberty with girls. Let's take a quick look at boys.

At puberty the sex hormones wake up in boys, and their increased production translates into a monumental transformation.

As a direct response to stimulation by the pituitary and hypothalamus glands in the brain, boys' hormones spring into action, just as in girls, and a series of significant changes occur that translate into adolescence.

Remember the Tanner Scale from chapter 4? The same scale applies to boys, following the development of their male bodies as seen from the outside in response to hormone stimulation on the inside. Body odor and voice changes, muscle and body organ growth, increasing height and weight—these are all characteristic changes the boy has to undergo in his transition to adulthood.

Tanner 1: No evidence of hair in armpits or pubis (prepuberty)

Tanner 2: Sparse armpit hair; thin pubic hair appears, covering a limited area of the pubis

Tanner 3: Increasing amounts of armpit hair; pubic hair coarser and more widely distributed in the pubic area; testicles and penis increasing in size; hair appearing on scrotum

Tanner 4: Pubic and armpit hair full and coarse; pubic hair doesn't reach the navel; penis and testicles nearing adult size

Tanner 5: Fully developed adult hair distribution in armpits, on pubis, and over body; full-size penis and testicles; adult voice

While these physical changes occur on the outside, on the inside the boys' testicles start to grow, and inside them sperm is produced. Testosterone, the main male-defining sex hormone, is released into the bloodstream. Testosterone precipitates the appearance of the physical changes described by the Tanner Scale. In addition, boys' muscles grow to adult size in direct response to the action of testosterone inside the body. Along with the testosterone, estrogen and progesterone are released to lesser extents.

Leptin, the hormone made by fat cells that rises right before girls start to menstruate, is also made in boys' fat cells. However, in direct opposition to its action in females, leptin production decreases to herald the beginning of puberty in boys. Boys who are overweight have been found to have higher levels of leptin and delayed puberty. Weight gain is not something that builds muscle mass and brings on puberty in boys.

My clinical experience with boys comes from fifteen years of being the school physician for the Irvington School District in Westchester County, New York. In my capacity as school physician, I followed hundreds of boys from elementary school through middle and finally high school. I performed school and sports physicals on them regularly and watched them transition from little boys into adult men. From the medical standpoint, I followed Tanner Scale guidelines when determining their qualification for sports and growth and development charts when evaluating their physical status.

From a human standpoint, I watched in amazement how in time the little boys went on to become young men.

Invariably I was faced with two common scenarios: little overweight boys who, with the approach of puberty, started to rapidly lose the weight and turn into athletic, muscle-bound young men, on the one hand; and on the other, little overweight boys who only became more overweight with the passage of time and who experienced a puberty that did not arrive as expected but rather was often significantly delayed for even years at a time.

Once attention was paid to the weight status of the latter group and they lost weight, puberty started catching up with them, and the usual transformations seen in their thinner counterparts soon followed.

Emotional Changes

Similar to the sudden changes in girls that occur with the release of sex hormones, boys also undergo significant emotional changes.

The boy's body image has to rapidly change to prepare for the male role of reproduction that emerges at adolescence.

Even though we as a society are not very well attuned to the emotional changes boys undergo, we need to acknowledge their presence if we are committed to helping them navigate this transitional period with minimal problems.

Historically boys have been subject to different types of stressors than girls. As aptly put by one of my patients: "Boys go to the school yard and have a fistfight to set their differences straight. Girls use gossip and mean words instead."

To be able to participate in the physical world of men, teen boys have to mature physically to become men. Today things are changing for boys as well.

With the increasing incidence of obesity in boys, new or newly noticed hormone problems are present in males. Obesity has been linked to delay in onset of puberty in boys. This is different than with girls, for whom increased weight has been connected to early puberty. The hormonal and emotional problems that arise from delayed puberty pose a different set of complications for males.

Overweight boys stay young longer, they don't mature, and their physical appearance does not develop—there's no armpit hair, no pubic hair, and no deepening voices, and testicles and penises remain small. The emotional fallout is very significant and often tragic. Ridicule and inability to compete with the high testosterone–driven boys keep the overweight boys in the background and away from competitive sports, physical enterprises, and girls.

While *The Teen Weight-Loss Solution* focuses on the problems overweight has on the hormones and lives of teen girls, we need to understand the issues of overweight teen boys as well. The solutions I would like you to use for your boys hinge primarily on the use of the same diet, exercise, and lifestyle changes you are now using to help your teen girls.

Hormone therapies in boys are not as well researched, and the few available studies are embryonic in their scope. Until we know more about how to hormonally balance our boys, let's start by becoming aware of their existence, and implementing the diet and exercise portions of *The Teen Weight-Loss Solution.*

Summary

Our teens are becoming more and more overweight. Almost daily we are exposed to new study results in articles or on television specials about the growing problem with teen obesity in our country.

Adolescent girls are encountering an onslaught of hormone problems as soon as they enter puberty, seemingly at earlier ages than in previous generations. Plagued with irregular periods, acne, mood swings, PMS, and weight gain, our young women are suffering while their mothers helplessly look on.

Scientific data are accumulating on the rising incidence of high cholesterol and increased risk of heart disease at younger ages. While research and public awareness in the areas of teen obesity, early puberty, and the long-term dangers posed by these problems to our adolescent daughters will continue to become more prominent in our lives, you and your daughter must have access to immediate solutions.

You cannot afford to become more confused and worried about your adolescent. You must be able to help her live her life successfully now.

The book you have just read offers you a combination of safe, commonsense, and scientific solutions you should start using today to help save your daughter.

There are no guarantees in life. I cannot tell you that by following my plan your daughter will become prom queen, get a full academic scholarship at an Ivy League school, or be recruited by the Ford modeling agency. I can assure you, however, that by following the solutions offered in this book, she will feel better about herself, she will lose weight and have fewer hormone problems, and she will become a healthier, happier, and more secure adult.

I promise you that there is light at the end of the teen tunnel and that you and your teen will see it clearly by the time you finish reading this book.

Appendix 1
Recipes

Make eating a family affair. The best way to help your teen is to work with her to develop healthy eating habits at home. Make eating fun and not the focus of a weight-control program. Meals should also be a way to spend quality time with your teen. Start with the following recipes and use them to cook together and have fun. You'll both lose weight, as well as create an environment where eating is not a source of stress.

BREAKFAST

TEX MEX TOFU SCRAMBLE

2 teaspoons canola oil

½ cup chopped red bell pepper

1 small jalapeño, seeded and finely diced (optional)

4 small corn tortillas

2 eggs

2 egg whites

⅛ teaspoon salt

⅛ teaspoon freshly ground pepper

1 cup soft tofu, drained and cut into small cubes

½ cup grated reduced-fat cheddar or Monterey Jack cheese

1 tablespoon chopped cilantro

1 cup canned reduced-fat refried beans, warmed in a microwave
   or over low heat

4 tablespoons store-bought tomato salsa

4 teaspoons reduced-fat sour cream for garnish

In a large nonstick sauté pan, over medium-high heat, add the oil, peppers, and jalapeño sauté until they are softened, about 2 to 3 minutes. Meanwhile, wrap the tortillas in a damp paper towel and microwave for 10 to 15 seconds, until they are warm and pliable.

In a small bowl, beat the eggs and egg whites with the salt and pepper. Add the tofu, cheese, and cilantro. Add to the sauté pan with the softened peppers and cook, stirring gently with a fork, until the eggs are softly scrambled.

Quickly spread the warm beans over each tortilla, add the egg mixture, and serve either open-faced or rolled up. Top with a tablespoon of salsa and a teaspoon of sour cream.

SERVES 4

BANANA NUT SPICE MUFFINS

This is a reduced-fat recipe.

1½ cups all-purpose flour

½ cup whole wheat flour

1 teaspoon cinnamon

⅛ teaspoon nutmeg

½ teaspoon salt

1 teaspoon baking soda

1 egg

3 ripe bananas, mashed

¾ cup light-brown sugar

1 teaspoon vanilla extract

¼ cup vegetable oil

½ cup chopped pecans or walnuts

Preheat the oven to 350°F. Grease a 12-cup muffin tin or line the tin with paper cups.

In a small bowl, whisk together the flours, cinnamon, nutmeg, salt, and baking soda to evenly combine. In a large bowl, whisk together the egg, bananas, sugar, vanilla, and oil until well combined.

Switch to a rubber spatula and gently fold the flour mixture into the banana mixture, taking care not to overstir. Fold in the chopped nuts. The batter will be lumpy. Gently spoon the batter into the muffin tins.

Bake for 25 to 30 minutes, or until a toothpick inserted into the center of the muffin comes out clean. Place on rack, let cool for 3 minutes, and remove muffins from tin.

MAKES 12 MUFFINS

SPINACH AND CHEESE STRATA

1 (10-ounce) package frozen spinach, thawed

2 tablespoons olive oil

1 large finely chopped onion

1 teaspoon salt

½ teaspoon black pepper

Pinch cayenne

¼ teaspoon freshly grated nutmeg

6 cups cubed French or Italian bread

1 cup feta cheese, crumbled

½ cup parmesan cheese, grated, plus extra for topping

2½ cups skim milk

3 eggs

3 egg whites

¼ teaspoon mustard

Grease a 9-by-13-inch baking pan or gratin dish with softened butter or vegetable spray.

Squeeze excess water from the spinach to remove as much liquid as possible, then finely chop. Heat the oil in a large sauté pan over medium-high heat and sauté the onion until soft, 4 to 5 minutes. Add half of the salt and pepper and add all of the cayenne, nutmeg, and spinach. Continue to cook for 1 minute, then remove from the heat.

Spread 2 cups of the bread cubes in the baking dish and top evenly with one-third of the spinach mixture. Sprinkle with one-third of each cheese. Repeat the layering twice more.

In a large bowl, whisk together the milk, eggs, egg whites, mustard, and the remaining salt and pepper and pour evenly over the strata. Cover with plastic wrap and refrigerate for at least 8 hours or overnight.

Preheat the oven to 350°F. Remove the strata from the refrigerator and let stand at room temperature for 30 minutes. Remove plastic wrap. Sprinkle top with a fine layer of Parmesan cheese.

Bake strata for 45 minutes, or until golden brown and puffy.

SERVES 6 TO 8

BERRY SMOOTHIE

½ cup fresh or frozen blueberries

½ cup fresh or frozen raspberries

1 ripe medium banana

¼ cup nonfat vanilla yogurt

¾ cup soy or skim milk

Pinch of cinnamon

Pinch of nutmeg

4 or 5 ice cubes

Place all ingredients in a blender and blend until smooth.

MAKES 1 LARGE SERVING

DESSERTS

CHOCOLATE, RASPBERRY, AND HAZELNUT PHYLLO PURSES

3 sheets phyllo dough

4 tablespoons unsalted butter, melted

4 ounces bittersweet chocolate

½ cup raspberries

¼ cup granulated sugar

2 tablespoons hazelnuts, skinned, toasted, and chopped (optional)

Preheat oven to 350°F.

On a cutting board or clean counter, lay out 1 sheet of phyllo dough. Brush it lightly with melted butter and place another sheet on top. Brush with more butter, then top with the third sheet. Cut the stacked sheets into four squares. Place 1 ounce of chocolate in the center of each square. Top with 3 or 4 raspberries. Gather the four corners of the phyllo square up around the chocolate and twist together to form a "purse." Repeat. Carefully transfer the purses to a baking sheet. Brush the purses with remaining butter and sprinkle with the sugar. Bake for 10 to 12 minutes, or until golden brown. Transfer to a plate and sprinkle with the hazelnuts.

SERVES 4

CARAMELIZED FRUIT AND HONEY YOGURT

1½ pounds assorted stone fruit, quartered, with stones removed
     (about 10 peaches, plums, nectarines, or apricots)
3 tablespoons butter, melted
¼ cup brown sugar
Frozen vanilla yogurt or plain low-fat yogurt, for serving

Preheat the oven to 400°F.

In a large well-buttered baking dish (ceramic or Pyrex work best) toss the prepared fruit with the melted butter and brown sugar. Bake for 20 minutes, stirring occasionally, or until the fruit is tender and slightly caramelized. Serve over a scoop of frozen yogurt or stirred into plain low-fat yogurt.

SERVES 4

HARVEST CRISP

2 large tart apples (such as Gravenstein), peeled, cored, and sliced
2 large pears, peeled, cored, and sliced
1 teaspoon ground cinnamon
¼ teaspoon ground nutmeg
¼ cup sugar
¾ cup flour
¾ cup packed dark-brown sugar

¾ cup old-fashioned oats

⅛ teaspoon salt

1½ sticks unsalted butter, cut into small pieces and chilled

¾ cup walnuts, chopped

Preheat oven to 350°F. Butter a ceramic or glass baking dish, such as a 14-inch oval casserole or 11-by-7-inch baking pan.

In a large bowl, combine the fruit, spices, and sugar, then place in baking dish.

In a bowl, combine the flour, brown sugar, oats, and salt. Cut in the butter with a pastry cutter or your fingertips until evenly distributed. Stir in the walnuts.

Spoon the topping over the fruit mixture. Bake 35 to 40 minutes, or until the juices bubble and the topping is golden brown.

SERVES 4

SNACKS

GRILLED BANANA NUTELLA PANINI

4 slices wheat bread or rustic country bread

½ cup Nutella spread (chocolate and hazelnut)

1 banana, thinly sliced

1 teaspoon butter or vegetable oil spray

Heat a panini press or an indoor grill pan or sauté pan over medium-high heat.

Grill the bread until toasted, about 1 minute. Spread half the Nutella over two slices of toast. Top the Nutella with banana slices and then top each with a second slice of toast. Butter both sides of the sandwiches, place in the panini press, and close the press and cook for 1 minute. If using a grill or sauté pan, press the sandwiches with a heavy pan.

SERVES 2

EDAMAME WITH CITRUS SALT

1 (1-pound) bag edamame
1 teaspoon seasoned citrus salt (or 1 teaspoon salt mixed with
    the zest of 2 lemons)

Bring a large pot of salted water to a boil. Prepare an ice-water bath and set aside. Add edamame to boiling water and boil for about 4 minutes, until bright green and just tender. Drain in a colander and add the edamame to the ice-water bath to stop the cooking. Drain again and toss with the seasoned salt.

SERVES 2

SPICED CURRY
OR CHILI POPCORN

1 bag low-fat microwave popcorn (preferably 94 percent
　　fat-free)

Vegetable spray

1 tablespoon curry powder or chili powder, or more to taste

Prepare popcorn according to the package directions. Place in very large bowl and spray once with vegetable spray. Quickly sprinkle with the curry or chili powder and toss to coat evenly.

SERVES 2

LUNCH OR DINNER

MEDITERRANEAN WRAP

2 zucchinis, cut into ½-inch dice

1 eggplant, cut into ½-inch dice

3 tablespoons olive oil

½ teaspoon salt

½ teaspoon pepper

4 rosemary or thyme sprigs

4 (10-inch) or larger flatbread rounds or flour tortillas

⅓ cup store-bought tapenade (black olive paste) or sun-dried
　　tomato spread

4 roasted red peppers in oil, drained, cut into slivers

1 (8-ounce) log goat cheese, crumbled

2 tablespoons chopped fresh mint

½ lemon, seeds removed

Preheat the oven to 425°F.

In a large bowl, toss the zucchini and eggplant with the oil, salt, pepper, and herb sprigs. Transfer the vegetables to a large roasting pan. Roast, shaking the pan often, for 15 to 20 minutes, until tender and slightly caramelized. Set aside and cool slightly.

Wrap the flatbreads together, flat, in damp paper towels and microwave for 15 seconds, or in additional 5-second bursts, or warm in a 200°F oven until pliable and warm.

Spread one-quarter of the tapenade over the entire surface of each flatbread. Top with roasted vegetables and the red peppers, goat cheese, and mint. Squeeze a little lemon juice over each serving. Season with salt and pepper. Gently tuck in the sides and tightly roll up the bread. Slice on the diagonal to serve.

SERVES 4

PASTA WITH CHICKEN SAUSAGE, SPINACH, AND WHITE BEANS

2 tablespoons extra-virgin olive oil

1 pound chicken or turkey sausage (not breakfast sausage),
    removed from casing

3 cloves garlic, crushed

1 small onion, finely chopped

1 can (28 to 32 ounces) chunky-style crushed tomatoes

1 (10-ounce) package frozen spinach, thawed and excess water
    removed

1 can cannellini beans, rinsed and drained

2 tablespoons fresh basil, chopped, or 2 teaspoons dried

1 pound penne rigate, cooked al dente

Pinch of hot Italian dried pepper, or more to taste

Salt and freshly ground black pepper

Grated Parmesan or Romano cheese, for serving

Heat the oil in a large sauté pan over medium-high heat. Add
the chicken or turkey sausage, stirring and breaking up the meat
as it browns. Add the garlic and onion and cook 5 minutes, stirring frequently. Reduce the heat to medium-low. Add the tomatoes, spinach, and beans and simmer 2 to 3 minutes, until
bubbling. Remove the pan from the heat and fold in the basil to
wilt. Place pasta in bowl, mix in sauce and hot pepper, and season with salt and pepper. Top with grated Parmesan or Romano
cheese and serve immediately.

SERVES 4

GREAT GRAIN SALAD
*This salad can be served warm alongside a roasted pork loin,
beef roast, or roasted chicken.*

3 tablespoons canola oil

½ cup chopped shallots

1 cup brown rice

1 cup wild rice

1 cup wheat berries

2 cups water

2 cups low-sodium chicken broth

½ cup balsamic vinegar

2 tablespoons extra-virgin olive oil

2 tablespoons chopped rosemary

½ teaspoon salt

¼ teaspoon freshly ground pepper

½ cup dried cranberries

½ cup chopped dried apricots

½ cup dried currants

1 cup coarsely chopped pecans, toasted

Heat the canola oil in large saucepan over medium-high heat. Add the shallots and sauté until translucent, about 5 minutes. Add the brown rice, wild rice, and wheat berries and stir to coat in oil. Add the water and stock and bring to a boil. Reduce the heat to low and cover. Cook until the grains are tender and the liquid is absorbed, about 40 minutes.

In a small bowl, whisk together the vinegar, olive oil, rosemary, salt, and pepper. Set aside.

Remove the grains from the heat. Stir in the dried cranberries, apricots, currants, and the dressing. Stir in the pecans. Season to taste with salt and pepper.

SERVES 4 TO 6

TURKEY CHILI

1 tablespoon olive oil

2 onions, chopped

2 pounds ground turkey

3 cloves garlic, minced

1 to 3 jalapeños (to taste), seeded and diced

½ teaspoon salt

1 teaspoon ground cumin

3 tablespoons chili powder

1 (28-ounce) can plum tomatoes, with liquid

3 cups low-sodium chicken broth or water

Sour cream, grated cheddar, and tortilla chips, for garnish

Heat the oil in a large saucepan or Dutch oven over medium-high heat. Add the onions and ground turkey, stirring often, until the turkey is just cooked through, about 5 minutes. Add the garlic, jalapeños, salt, cumin, and chili powder and sauté for another 1 to 2 minutes, taking care not to burn the garlic.

Add the tomatoes and broth, reduce the heat to low, and simmer for 45 minutes to an hour, until the sauce is slightly thickened. Serve over rice and garnish with sour cream, grated cheddar, and tortilla chips.

SERVES 6

CRUNCHY ASIAN CHICKEN SALAD

If you don't have time to make the dressings,

you can use store-bought sesame-ginger dressing.

¾ cup crispy chow mein noodles, plus additional noodles for
    garnish

3 cups shredded cooked chicken, without skin (from a rotisserie
    chicken or a cooked breast)

¼ cup dry-roasted, unsalted cashews

1 cup minced fresh coriander

1 red bell pepper, cut into julienne strips

1 bunch of scallions, cut into 1-inch pieces

1 cup bean sprouts

3 cups green cabbage, shredded

2 romaine hearts, cut into chiffonade

For the dressing

½ teaspoon dry mustard

1 tablespoon soy sauce

3 tablespoons rice wine vinegar

2 tablespoons hoisin sauce

1 teaspoon freshly grated ginger

1 teaspoon sugar

Salt and fresly ground pepper

2 tablespoons sesame oil

¼ cup canola oil

In a large bowl, combine the crispy noodles, chicken, cashews, coriander, bell pepper, scallions, sprouts, cabbage, and romaine.

For the dressing, whisk together the mustard, soy sauce, vinegar, hoisin sauce, ginger, sugar, and salt and pepper to taste. Whisk in the oils in a stream, emulsifying the dressing.

Toss the chicken salad with enough dressing to coat, and garnish with additional crispy noodles.

SERVES 6 GENEROUSLY

FISH TACOS

1½ pounds cod or snapper fillets

Salt and freshly ground black pepper

2 teaspoons canola oil

1 cup seeded and chopped tomatoes (about ½ pound)

1 red onion, diced

3 scallions, thinly sliced

2 fresh jalapeños, seeded and minced (or to taste)

2 tablespoons fresh lime juice

2 tablespoons white wine vinegar

3 tablespoons olive oil

3 tablespoons chopped fresh coriander

2 cups romaine lettuce or green cabbage, shredded

12 (6-inch) corn tortillas

Season the fillets with salt and pepper. Heat the canola oil in a large sauté pan over medium-high heat and sear the fish on each side. Reduce the heat to low, cover, and cook until opaque, 2 to 3 minutes, depending on the thickness of the fillets.

To make the filling, in a bowl toss together the fish, tomatoes, red onion, scallions, jalapeños, lime juice, vinegar, olive oil, coriander, and salt and pepper. Chill the filling, covered, for at least one hour or overnight.

Wrap the tortillas in a damp paper towel and microwave for 15 seconds, or until warm and pliable. Top each tortilla with shredded romaine or cabbage and top with fish. Serve with store-bought refried beans and rice.

SERVES 4 TO 6

SEARED SALMON WITH MANGO SALSA

3 tablespoons ancho chile powder

2 tablespoons kosher salt

2 tablespoons black pepper

4 salmon fillets or steaks, about 6 ounces each

Olive oil

Mango Salsa (recipe follows)

Preheat an outdoor grill to medium or heat an indoor grill to medium-high. (A sauté pan will work as well.)

In a small bowl, mix together the ancho chile powder, salt, and pepper.

Brush both sides of the fillets or steaks with olive oil and rub the chile mixture on the flesh side of the fillets. Rub the chile mixture on both sides if using steaks. Place each fillet flesh side down on the hot grill and cook for about 3 minutes. Turn over and cook for an additional 3 to 5 minutes, until just opaque. Remove from the grill and top with mango salsa.

SERVES 4

Mango Salsa

2 mangoes, cut into small dice

1 medium red onion, finely diced

2 jalapeño peppers, minced

¼ cup chopped cilantro leaves

2 limes, juiced

2 tablespoons olive oil

Salt and freshly ground pepper

Mix all the ingredients together and chill.

MINESTRONE WITH PESTO SWIRL

2 teaspoons olive oil

1 yellow onion, finely diced

1 stalk celery, cut into ¼-inch pieces

2 carrots, peeled and cut into ½-inch pieces

3 garlic cloves, minced

¾ teaspoon freshly ground pepper

3 tablespoons finely chopped fresh oregano (or 1 teaspoon dried)

2 tablespoons finely chopped fresh thyme (or 2 teaspoons dried)

1 tablespoon finely chopped fresh rosemary

1 large eggplant, cut into ½-inch pieces

1 red bell pepper, cut into ½-inch pieces

1 zucchini (about 8 ounces), cut into ½-inch pieces

8 cups chicken broth (low-sodium canned is fine), skimmed of fat

2 (14½-ounce) cans whole peeled tomatoes

1 cup canned cannellini beans, drained and rinsed

¾ cup small pasta shells, cooked according to package directions

Pesto (store-bought), for garnish (optional)

Parmesan cheese, for garnish (optional)

In a stockpot, over medium heat, heat the oil. Add the onion, celery, carrots, garlic, pepper, oregano, thyme, and rosemary and sauté, stirring frequently, until the onions are soft and translucent, 5 to 8 minutes.

Add the eggplant, bell pepper, and zucchini and sauté until the vegetables are softened, about 5 minutes more. Add the chicken broth and tomatoes and bring to a boil, stirring to break up the tomatoes. Reduce the heat to low and let simmer until the vegetables are tender, 10 to 12 minutes. Add the beans and pasta and cook until heated through, about 2 minutes more. Swirl a teaspoon of pesto into each serving, and sprinkle with cheese.

SERVES 6 TO 8

BUTTERNUT AND APPLE SOUP WITH CURRIED YOGURT

8 cups (about 2 pounds) butternut squash, peeled and cut into
    large cubes

2 tablespoons olive oil

¾ cup plain low-fat yogurt

1 teaspoon curry powder

Salt and freshly ground pepper

1 tablespoon butter

2 cups peeled and chopped Granny Smith apples

1½ cups finely chopped onion

½ cup finely chopped celery

1 garlic clove, minced

3 (14½-ounce) cans fat-free, low-sodium chicken broth

½ teaspoon cinnamon

Preheat the oven to 400°F.

On a foil-lined baking sheet, toss the squash with 1 table-spoon of the olive oil. Arrange the squash in a single layer and bake for 45 minutes or until tender.

In a small bowl, mix the yogurt with the curry powder and season to taste with salt and pepper. Set aside.

In a large saucepan or stockpot, heat the remaining 1 table-spoon oil and the butter over medium-high heat. Add the apples, onions, celery, and garlic and sauté for 10 minutes. Add the roasted squash, chicken broth, cinnamon, ¼ teaspoon salt, and pepper and stir well. Reduce heat to medium-low and simmer, uncovered, for 30 minutes.

Partially mash the mixture with a potato masher until thick

and chunky, or puree in a food processor for a smoother consistency. Top each serving with a spoon of curried yogurt and freshly ground pepper.

SERVES 4

MEXICAN SHRIMP AND CORN SOUP

2½ tablespoons vegetable oil

4 (6-inch) corn tortillas, cut into ¼-inch strips (crumbled store-bought tortilla chips are okay)

2 cups corn kernels (4 ears if fresh)

1 cup finely diced red bell pepper

1½ teaspoons ground cumin

1 teaspoon dried oregano

2 garlic cloves, minced

2 jalapeño peppers, seeded and minced

½ cup thinly sliced scallions

2 cups diced tomatoes, fresh or canned

2 cups low-sodium chicken broth

1 cup bottled clam juice

1½ pounds medium shrimp, peeled and deveined

¼ cup chopped fresh cilantro

¼ cup freshly squeezed lime juice

⅛ teaspoon salt

¼ teaspoon pepper

Heat 1 tablespoon of the oil in a large Dutch oven or stockpot over medium-high heat. Add the tortilla strips and sauté 4 min-

utes or until crisp. Remove the strips and drain on paper towels.

Add ½ tablespoon of the oil to pan and heat. Add the corn and bell pepper and sauté until the corn is lightly golden brown, about 3 minutes. Add the cumin, oregano, garlic, jalapeños, and scallions and sauté for 2 minutes, stirring frequently. Add the tomatoes, chicken broth, and clam juice and bring to a boil. Reduce the heat and simmer 5 minutes.

Heat the remaining 1 tablespoon oil in a small sauté pan over high heat and sear the shrimp on each side. Continue to cook until opaque, about 3 minutes.

Remove the soup from heat, add the shrimp, and stir in the cilantro, lime juice, salt, and pepper. Ladle the soup into bowls. Divide the tortilla strips evenly over each serving.

SERVES 6

Appendix 2

Dr. Erika's Daily Journal

www.drerika.com

Today's Date: _____   Day of Cycle: _____
(Day 1 = Start of Period)

DIET

BREAKFAST	TIME	AMOUNT	FOOD BRAND

LUNCH	TIME	AMOUNT	FOOD BRAND

DINNER	TIME	AMOUNT	FOOD BRAND

SNACKS	TIME	AMOUNT	FOOD BRAND

LIQUIDS	TIME	AMOUNT	FOOD BRAND

EXERCISE

	GYM	SWIMMING	TEAM SPORT	AEROBIC	OTHER
TIME SPENT					

LIFESTYLE—HOW DO YOU FEEL TODAY?

	SATISFYING	REWARDING	EXCITING	STRESSFUL	BORED	TENSE
SCHOOL/WORK						
FRIENDS						
SIBLINGS						
PARENTS						

SLEEP

Number of hours _____ Continuous _____ Interrupted _____
Time you went to sleep _____

STRESS LEVEL

Rate 1–5 (1 = Minimum, 5 = Maximum): _____

SUPPLEMENTS (Circle what you took today)

L. Carnitine   Natural Progesterone?
Coenzyme Q_{10} _____ Yes _____ No
Omega-3
Multivitamin
Combination

Overall Rating of the Day (1–5): _____(1 = Excellent, 5 = Poor)

Glossary

Adrenarche Time in the development of the girl when pubic hair and body odor appear as a result of an increase in sex hormone production by the adrenal gland.

Androgens A number of masculinizing hormones present in both the male and female bodies that cause the growth of pubic and armpit (axillary) hair as well as an increase in male sexual organ size.

Androstenediol An androgenic (masculinizing) hormone made in the ovaries and adrenals that can be metabolized in fatty tissues into the estrogens estradiol, estriol, or estrone or be converted into testosterone.

Bioidentical   Bioidentical hormones also known as natural hormones are physiologically and chemically identical to human hormones. The molecules that make up bioidentical hormones are identical to human hormone molecules. They are usually derived from plant sources.

Birth control pills   (oral contraceptives, contraceptive patches, and contraceptive deposits) A group of synthetic hormones used to override the natural hormone cycle of the female body. Birth control pills are used as a contraceptive to prevent ovulation. They are also used to override the system in teens with irregular menstrual cycles.

Body mass index (BMI)   A measure of the amount of body fat that is calculated by dividing the height in meters squared by the weight in kilograms.

Cervix   The narrow outer end of the uterus that protrudes into the vagina.

Corpus luteum   Progesterone-secreting organ that develops from the follicle at the site of extrusion of the egg from the ovary at ovulation.

Cortisol   A steroid hormone produced by the adrenal gland. Cortisol is essential for the utilization of carbohydrates, fats, and proteins for a normal response to stress.

DHEA   Abbreviation for adrenal-produced androgen dihydroepiandrosterone. A precursor of testosterone.

Endocrine   Referring to the ductless glands (such as the thyroid, parathyroid, pituitary, thalamus, etc.) or tissue that produce hormones that are carried as messengers in the bloodstream.

Endometrium   The nutrient-rich mucous membrane lining the uterus. It is shed during menstruation or serves as support for the fertilized egg during initial stages of pregnancy.

Estradiol   Also known as E_2, the main human estrogen produced in the ovaries that is most abundant in teenagers and young adults.

Estriol   Also known as E_3; an estrogen that is a relatively weak metabolite of estradiol; produced in larger quantities in the body during pregnancy.

Estrogen   The name for the group of hormones that have feminizing effects in the body; sex hormones made in the ovaries, adrenals, and fat cells that promote female secondary sex characteristics: breast development, menstruation, mood, weight balance, and ovulation, among many other functions. Estrogen works in conjunction with all other hormones to provide hormonal and overall balance.

Fertility   In women, the ability to become pregnant; having the capability to produce offspring.

Follicle   The area in the ovary that protects and supports the maturation of the egg before ovulation.

Follicular phase   The first phase of the menstrual cycle following menstruation when follicles are starting to develop in the ovary, allowing for egg maturation prior to ovulation; also described as the proliferative phase.

FSH (follicle-stimulating hormone)   Hormone secreted by the anterior pituitary gland that stimulates development of the ovarian follicles, the maturation of the egg and sperm, and the production of estrogen.

GnRH (gonadotropin-releasing hormone)   A hormone produced by the hypothalamus gland sent to the pituitary, prompting the release of either FSH or LH (luteinizing hormone).

Gonadotropins   The LH (luteinizing) and FSH (follicle-stimulating hormone) hormones. Heralders of puberty produced by the pituitary gland that stimulate the ovaries and testes to start making estrogen, progesterone, and testosterone and turn a girl or boy into an adolescent.

Gonads   Reproductive glands (ovaries and testes).

Growth hormone (GH)   A hormone produced by the pituitary gland essential for growth and metabolism. GH levels drop after adolescence.

Hormone   The body's messengers; substances produced by cells that circulate in the bloodstream and body fluids and affect the actions of every cell and organ in the body.

Insulin   Hormone made in the pancreas with the function of lowering blood glucose levels and sending glucose for storage into the liver, muscle, and fat cells for later use.

Insulin-resistance A situation where the body does not respond to insulin and thus maintains high blood sugar levels. More insulin must be produced to bring sugar levels to normal. This is commonly seen in overweight people and is also considered a symptom of polycystic ovary disease. Weight reduction is often found to eliminate symptoms of insulin-resistance.

Leptin A hormone made by fat cells that is necessary to regulate body weight and enable puberty progression. Rise in leptin levels precipitates puberty in girls, drop in leptin precipitates puberty in boys.

LH (luteinizing hormone) A hormone secreted by the anterior pituitary gland that stimulates the ovaries and testes to make more hormones and prompts ovulation.

Lupron The brand name of the main drug used in the United States to prevent precocious puberty from progressing. One of its numerous side effects is weight gain. Long-term effects on adults who received Lupron as children are unknown.

Luteal phase The late phase of the menstrual cycle following ovulation when the corpus luteum significantly increases secretion of progesterone.

Mammography An X-ray of the breast; used to detect cancer and other abnormalities.

Menarche The time of the first menstrual period experienced by a girl.

Menopause   The normal cessation of the menstrual cycle in women, occurring usually in the late forties and early fifties. Clinically defined as when a woman has not had a period for a year.

Menstrual cycle   The changes that take place in a woman's body over the time span between the end of menstruation and the beginning of another menstruation. Physiologically includes: follicular, ovulation, and luteal phases.

Metabolism   The sum of all the physical and chemical processes occurring in the body.

Ovaries   The pair of female reproductive organs on either side of the lower abdomen or belly that produce eggs and secrete sex hormones: estrogen, progesterone, and testosterone.

Ovulation   The release of an egg from the ovarian follicle fourteen days before the beginning of a menstrual cycle; the point in time when fertilization can occur.

PCOs (polycystic ovary syndrome)   A constellation of symptoms including ovarian cysts, increased body hair, high testosterone levels, insulin-resistance, and obesity. In recent years, with the increase in weight problems and irregular menstruation in many teens, the diagnosis is made more frequently. Successful treatment is often found in changes in diet, weight loss, increase in exercise, and lifestyle changes.

Phytohormone   Hormones found in plants that exert hormone-like effects in the human body.

Pituitary gland   The endocrine gland located in the brain that produces FSH, LH, GH—all sex-organ stimulating hormones.

PMS (premenstrual syndrome)   A galaxy of symptoms experienced primarily but not exclusively in the days leading up to menstruation include but are not limited to: moodiness, irritability, headaches, bloating, increase or loss of appetite, food cravings, changes in bowel habits (constipation or diarrhea), sleep disturbance, and increased fatigue.

Progesterone   A female sex hormone secreted by the corpus luteum that helps prepare the lining of the uterus for the implantation of the egg. Progesterone is crucial to balance the negative effects of estrogen in a hormone supplementation regimen.

Systemic   Affecting the whole body function.

Tanner Scale   A method of categorizing a teen's stage of physical development commonly used in U.S. schools and pediatricians' offices, ranging from stage 1 (prepuberty: no breast or pubic hair development) to stage 5 (adult breast, pubic hair, and genitalia development).

Testosterone   A sex hormone that exists in smaller quantities in females and is dominant in males. It is responsible for sperm production, movement, and quality, and secondary sexual characteristics in males—body odor, hair, size of testicles and penis, muscle development, and certain personality traits identified with males (aggression, assertiveness, confrontation). In women testosterone is associated with increased energy, stamina, aggression, assertiveness, improved muscle building ability, increased facial and body hair.

Ultrasound　　A noninvasive radiologic test that uses sound to create images of internal organs like the ovaries and uterus without the danger of X-ray exposure.

Uterus　　The organ in the female body located in the abdomen under the pelvic bone. Its function is to house the fertilized egg and allow the embryo to develop. The lining of the uterus, called the endometrium, is sloughed off during menstruation, causing occasional "clots" and bleeding to occur.

Vitamins　　Organic compounds that help perform specific metabolic functions. The body cannot make vitamins, so they are obtained from the diet or from supplementation.

Recommended Readings and Resources

BOOKS

Dillard, Annie. *An American Childhood*. New York: Harper & Row, 1988.

Emans, J. H., and D. P. Goldstein. *Pediatric and Adolescent Gynecology*, 4th ed. Boston: Little, Brown, 1998.

Kaplowitz, Paul, M.D., Ph.D. *Early Puberty in Girls*. New York: Ballantine Books, 2004.

Neinstein, Laurence S., ed. *Adolescent Health Care: A Practical Guide*. Philadelphia: Lippincott, Williams and Wilkins, 2002.

Northrup, Christiane. *The Wisdom of Menopause*. New York: Bantam, 2001.

Pipher, May. *Reviving Ophelia: Saving the Selves of Adolescent Girls*. New York: Ballantine Books, 1994.

Rogers, Carl. *On Becoming a Person: A Therapist's View of Psychotherapy*. Boston: Houghton Mifflin, 1961.

Schwartz, Erika, M.D. *Natural Energy*. New York: Putnam, 1999.

———. *The Hormone Solution*. New York: Warner Books, 2002.

————. *The 30-Day Natural Hormone Plan.* New York: Warner Books, 2004.

Snyderman, Nancy, M.D., and Peg Streep. *Girl in the Mirror: Mothers and Daughters in Adolescence.* New York: Hyperion, 2002.

Waterston, Ellen. *Then There Was No Mountain: The Parallel Odyssey of a Mother and Daughter Through Addiction.* Lanham, Md.: Roberts Rinehart, 2003.

Wolf, Naomi. *The Beauty Myth: How Images of Beauty Are Used Against Women.* New York: Anchor Books, 1992.

NEWSPAPER AND MAGAZINE ARTICLES

Ball, Deborah. "Swedish Kids Show Difficulty of Fighting Fat." *Wall Street Journal,* December 2, 2003.

Brody, Jane. "Personal Health: Yesterday's Precocious Puberty Is Norm Today." *New York Times,* November 30, 1999.

Goode, Erica. "How to Talk to Teenage Girls About Weight? Very Carefully." *New York Times,* June 26, 2003.

Gorman, Christine. "Why Are So Many of Us Getting Diabetes?" *Time,* December 8, 2003.

————. "Desperate Measures." *Time,* November 17, 2003.

Hoffmann, Bill. "America's Tubby Teens Top the Scales." *New York Post,* January 6, 2004.

Kalb, Claudia. "Troubled Souls." *Newsweek,* September 22, 2003.

Kantrowitz, Barbara, and Karen Springen. "Why Sleep Matters." *Newsweek,* September 22, 2003.

Kolata, Gina. "Just How Low Can You Go? A Cholesterol Challenge." *New York Times,* December 2, 2003.

Tanner, Lindsey (Associated Press). "Study Says U.S. Teens Are Fattest." *Star Telegram,* January 5, 2004.

Tyre, Peg, and Julie Scelfo. "Helping Kids Get Fit." *Newsweek,* September 22, 2003.

Villarosa, Linda. "Prevention Can Start Young, Studies Suggest; But How?" *New York Times,* December 2, 2003.

Woolf, Alan, M.D., M.P.H., and Leann Lesperance, M.D., Ph.D. "What Should We Worry About?" *Newsweek,* September 22, 2003.

SURVEYS AND STUDIES

White House Office of National Drug Control Policy (John P. Walters, director). "Teen Drug Abuse Declines Across Wide Front." Monitoring the Future Survey, December 19, 2003.

SCHOLARLY ARTICLES

Abramowitz, Beth, M.S., and Leann Birch, Ph.D. "Five-Year-Old Girls' Ideas About Dieting Are Predicted by Mothers' Dieting." *Journal of the American Dietetic Association* 100, no. 10 (October 2000).

Alderman, E. M. "Breast Problems in the Adolescent." *Patient Care* 30 (March 2000): 56–80.

Alton, I. R. "Nutritional Needs and Assessment of Adolescents." In *Adolescent Health Care,* edited by R. W. Blum. New York: Academic Press, 1982.

Anderson, S. E., G. E. Dallal, and A. Must. "Relative Weight and Race Influence Average Age at Menarche: Results from Two Nationally Representative Surveys of U.S. Girls Twenty-five Years Apart." *Pediatrics* 111 (2003): 844–50.

Angell, M., and J. P. Kassirer. "Alternative Medicine: The Risks of Untested and Unregulated Remedies." *New England Journal of Medicine* 339, no. 12 (1998): 839–41.

Anstin, D., and D. Grinenko. "Rapid Screening for Disordered Eating in College-aged Females in the Primary Care Setting." *Journal of Adolescent Health* 26 (2000): 338.

Barash, I. A., C. C. Cheung, D. S. Weigle, et al. "Leptin Is a Metabolic Signal to the Reproductive System." *Endocrinology* 137 (1996): 3144–47.

Bauer, B. S., K. M. Jones, and C. W. Talbot. "Mammary Masses in the Adolescent Female." *Gynecology and Obstetrics Surgery* 165 (1987): 63.

Borrud L., C. Wilkinson Enns, and S. Mickle. "What We Eat: USDA Surveys Food Consumption Changes." *Institute of Community Nutrition* (1997): 4.

Braet, C. "Treatment of Obese Children: A New Rationale." *Clinical Child Psychology and Psychiatry* 4 (1999): 579.

Brill, S. R., and W. D. Rosenfeld. "Contraception." *Medical Clinics of North America* 84 (2000): 907.

Centers for Diseases Control and Prevention. "Prevalence of Overweight Among Children, Adolescents, and Adults: United States, 1988–1994." *Morbidity and Mortality Weekly Report* 46 (1997): 199. Available at www.cdc.gov/epo/mmwr/preview/mmwrhtml/00046647.htm.

———. "Trends in Sexual Risk Behaviors Among High School Students, United States, 1991–1997." *Morbidity and Mortality Weekly Report* 47 (1998): 749.

Clarkson, P. M. "Nutrition for Improved Sports Performance: Current Issues on Ergogenic Aids." *Sports Medicine* 21 (1996): 393.

Committee to Develop Criteria for Evaluating the Outcomes of Approaches to Prevent and Treat Obesity, Food and Nutrition Board, Institute of Medicine, National Academy of Sciences. "Summary: Weighing the Options—Criteria for Evaluating Weight-Management Programs." *Journal of the American Dietetic Association* 95 (1995): 96.

Daniles, S. R., P. R. Khoury, and J. A. Morrison. "The Utility of Body Mass Index as a Measure of Body Fatness in Children and Adolescents: Differences by Race and Gender." *Pediatrics* 99 (1997): 804–7.

Davtyan, C. "Evidence-Based Case Review: Contraception for Adolescents." *Western Journal of Medicine* 172 (2000): 166.

Denke, M. A., C. T. Sempos, and S. M. Grundy. "Excess Body Weight: An Underrecognized Contributor to Dyslipidemia in White American Women." *Archives of Internal Medicine* 154 (1994): 401.

Dietz, W. D. "Therapeutic Strategies in Childhood Obesity." *Hormone Research* 39 (1993): 86.

Dudgeon, D. L. "Pediatric Breast Lesions: Take the Conservative Approach." *Contemporary Pediatrics* (January 1985): 61–73.

Dunger, D. B., and M. A. Preece. "Growth and Nutrient Requirements at Adolescence." In *Pediatric Nutrition: Theory and Practice,* edited by R. J. Grand, J. L. Sutphen, and W. H. Dietz Jr. Boston: Butterworths, 1987.

Facchinetti, F., A. D. Genazzani, E. Martignoni, et al. "Neuroendocrine Changes in Luteal Function in Patients with Premenstrual Syndrome." *Journal of Clinical Endocrinology and Metabolism* 76 (1993): 1123.

Firenzuoli, F., and L. Gori. "Garcinia Cambogia for Weight Loss." *Journal of the American Medical Association* 282 (1999): 234.

"Fish Oil May Help Relieve Depression." *Internal Medicine World Report* (December 2002): A12–31.

Ford, C. A., S. G. Millstein, B. L. Halpern-Felsher, et al. "Influence of Physician Confidentiality Assurances on Adolescents' Willingness to Disclose Information and Seek Future Health Care: A Randomized Controlled Trial." *Journal of the American Medical Association* 278 (1997): 1029.

Freedman, D. S., L. K. Khan, M. K. Serdula, et al. "Relation of Menarche to Race, Time Period, and Anthropomorphic Dimensions: The Bogalusa Heart Study." *Pediatrics* 110 (2002): e43.

Freeman, E. W., K. Rickels, S. J. Sondheimer, et al. "A Double-blind Trial of Oral Progesterone, Alprazolam, and Placebo in Treatment of Severe Premenstrual Syndrome." *Journal of the American Medical Association* 274 (1995): 51.

Frisch, R. E., and J. W. McArthur. "Menstrual Cycles: Fatness as a Determinant of Minimum Weight for Height Necessary for Their Maintenance and Onset." *Science* 185 (1974): 949–51.

Gross, I., M. Wheeler, and K. Hess. "The Treatment of Obesity in Adolescents Using Behavioral Self-control." *Clinical Pediatrics* (Philadelphia) 15 (1976): 920.

Hacker, K. A., Y. Amare, N. Strunk, et al. "Listening to Youth: Teen Perspectives on Pregnancy Prevention." *Journal of Adolescent Health* 26 (2000): 279.

Halbreich, U. "Premenstrual Syndromes: Closing the Twentieth-Century Chapters." *Current Opinions in Obstetrics and Gynecology* 11 (1999): 265.

He, Q., and J. Karlberg. "BMI Gain in Childhood and Its Association with Height Gain, Timing of Puberty, and Final Height." *Pediatric Research* 49 (2001): 244–51.

Herbold, N., and S. Frates. "Update of Nutrition Guidelines for the Teen Trends and Concerns." *Current Opinions in Pediatrics* 12 (2000): 303.

Hergenroeder, A. C., and S. Phillips. "Advising Teenagers and Young Adults About Weight Gain and Loss Through Exercise and Diet: Practical Advice for the Physician." In *Monographs in Clinical Pediatrics: Adolescent Medicine,* edited by I. R. Shenker, pp. 133–36. Chur, Switz.: Harwood Academic, 1994.

Herman-Giddens, M. E., E. J. Slora, R. C. Wasserman, et al. "Secondary Sexual Characteristics and Menses in Young Girls Seen in Office Practice: A Study from the Pediatrics Research in Office Settings Network." *Pediatrics* 99 (1997): 505–12.

Heymsfield, S. B., A. S. Greenberg, K. Fujioka, et al. "Recombinant Leptin for Weight Loss in Obese and Lean Adults: A Randomized, Controlled, Dose-Escalation Trial." *Journal of the American Medical Association* 282 (1999): 1568.

Hill, J., and J. Peters. "Environmental Contributions to the Obesity Epidemic." *Science* 280 (1998): 1371.

Himes, J. H., and W. D. Dietz. "Guidelines for Overweight in Adolescent Preventive Services: Recommendations from an Expert Committee." *American Journal of Clinical Nutrition* 59 (1994): 307.

Hulanicka, B., L. Gronkiewicz, and J. Koniarek. "Effect of Familial Distress on Growth and Maturation of Girls: A Longitudinal Study." *American Journal of Human Biology* 13 (2001): 771–76.

Kann, L., S. A. Kinchen, B. I. Williams, et al. "Youth Risk Behavior Surveillance: United States, 1997." *Morbidity and Mortality Weekly Report* 47 (1998): 1.

Kaplowitz, P. B., S. E. Oberfield, and the Drug and Therapeutics and Executive Committees of the Lawson Wilkins Pediatric Endocrine Society. "Reexamination of the Age Limit for Defining When Puberty Is Precocious in Girls in the United States: Implications for Evaluation and Treatment." *Pediatrics* 104 (1999): 936–41.

Kendall, K. E., and P. P. Schnurr. "The Effects of Vitamin B$_6$ Supplementation on Premenstrual Symptoms." *Obstetrics and Gynecology* 70 (1987): 145.

Klein, J. R., and I. F. Litt. "Epidemiology of Adolescent Dysmenorrhea." *Pediatrics* 68 (1981): 661.

Lin-Su, K., M. G. Vogiatsi, and M. I. New. "Body Mass Index and Age at Menarche in an Adolescent Clinic Population." *Clinical Pediatrics* 41 (2002): 501–7.

Lloyd, T., M. B. Andon, N. Rollis, et al. "Calcium Supplementation and Bone Mineral Density in Adolescent Girls." *Journal of the American Medical Association* 270 (1993): 841–44.

Mokdad, A. H., M. K. Serdula, and W. H. Dietz. "The Spread of the Obesity Epidemic in the United States, 1991–1998." *Journal of the American Medical Association* 282 (1999): 1519.

Must, A., J. Spandano, E. H. Coakley, et al. "The Disease Burden Associated with Overweight and Obesity." *Journal of the American Medical Association* 282 (1999): 1523.

National Heart, Lung, and Blood Institute, National Institutes of Health. "Clinical Guidelines on the Identification, Evaluation, and Treatment of Overweight and Obesity in Adults (executive summary)." *Archives of Internal Medicine* 158 (1998): 1855.

National Task Force on the Prevention and Treatment of Obesity. "Very Low-Calorie Diets." *Journal of the American Medical Association* 270 (1993): 967.

O'Brien, P. M. "Helping Young Women with Premenstrual Syndrome." *British Medical Journal* 307 (1993): 1471.

O'Brien, P. M., K. Wyatt, and P. Dimmock. "Premenstrual Syndrome Is Real and Treatable." *Practitioner* 244 (2000): 185.

Ogden, C. L., K. M. Flegal, M. D. Carroll, and C. L. Johnson. "Prevalence and Trends in Overweight Among U.S. Children and Adolescents, 1999–2000." *Journal of the American Medical Association* 288 (2002): 1728–32.

Overpeck, Mary, Ph.D., and Mary Hediger, Ph.D. "Teenagers in the U.S. Have Higher Rates of Obesity Than Those in Fourteen Other Industrialized Countries." *Archives of Pediatrics and Adolescent Medicine* (January 5, 2004).

Paige, D. M. "Obesity in Childhood and Adolescence." *Postgraduate Medicine* 79 (1986): 233.

Paretsch, C.-J., and W. G. Sippell. "Pathogenesis and Epidemiology of Precocious Puberty: Effects of Exogenous Oestrogens." *Human Reproduction Update* 7 (2001): 292–302.

Parker, P. D. "Premenstrual Syndrome." *American Family Physician* 50 (1994): 1309.

Pearlstein, T. B. "Hormones and Depression: What Are the Facts About Premenstrual Syndrome, Menopause, and Hormone Replacement Therapy?" *American Journal of Obstetrics and Gynecology* 173 (1995): 646.

Pedron-Nuevo, N., L. N. Gonzalez-Unzaga, R. De Celis-Carrillo, et al. "Incidence of Dysmenorrhea and Associated Symptoms in Women Aged Thirteen to Twenty-four Years." *Ginecologia e Obstetrica Mexicana* 66 (1998): 492.

Pietrobelli, A., M. Faith, D. Allison, et al. "Body Mass Index as a Measure of Adiposity Among Children and Adolescents: A Validation Study." *Journal of Pediatrics* 132 (1998): 204.

Racchinetti, F., P. Borella, G. Sauces, et al. "Oral Magnesium Successfully Relieves Premenstrual Mood Changes." *Obstetrics and Gynecology* 78 (1991): 177.

Ramcharan, S., F. A. Pellegrin, R. M. Ray, et al. "The Walnut Creek Contraceptive Drug Study: A Comprehensive Study of the Side Effects of Oral Contraception," vol. 3, "An Interim Report: A Comparison of Disease Occurrence Leading to Hospitalization or Death in

Users and Non-users of Oral Contraceptives." NIH Publication 81–54. Washington, D.C.: National Institutes of Health, 1981.

Rand, C. S., and A. M. Macgregor. "Adolescents Having Obesity Surgery: A Six-Year Follow-up." *Southern Medicine Journal* 87 (1994): 1208.

Ravussin, E., S. Lillioja, W. C. Knowler, et al. "Reduced Rate of Energy Expenditure as a Risk Factor for Body-Weight Gain." *New England Journal of Medicine* 318 (1988): 467.

Revicki, D. A., and R. G. Israel. "Relationship Between Body Mass Indices and Measures of Body Adiposity." *American Journal of Public Health* 76 (1986): 992.

Rieder, J., and S. M. Coupey. "The Use of Nonhormonal Methods of Contraception in Adolescents." *Pediatric Clinics of North America* 46 (1999): 671.

Robinson, T. N. "Defining Obesity in Children and Adolescents: Clinical Approaches." *Critical Review of Food Science Nutrition* 33 (1993): 313.

———. "Reducing Children's Television Viewing to Prevent Obesity: A Randomized Controlled Trial." *Journal of the American Medical Association* 282 (1999): 1561.

Robinson, T. N., L. D. Hammer, J. D. Killen, et al. "Does Television Viewing Increase Obesity and Reduce Physical Activity? Cross-sectional and Longitudinal Analyses Among Adolescent Girls." *Pediatrics* 91 (1993): 273.

Rocchini, A. P. "Adolescent Obesity and Hypertension." *Pediatric Clinics of North America* 40 (1993): 81.

Roseblatt, E. "Weight-Loss Programs: Pluses and Minuses of Commercial and Self-help Groups." *Postgraduate Medicine* 83 (1988): 137.

Rosner, B., R. Prineas, J. Loggie, and S. R. Daniels. "Percentiles for Body Mass Index in U.S. Children Five to Seventeen Years of Age." *Journal of Pediatrics* 132 (1998): 211–22.

Rumpel, C., and T. B. Harris. "The Influence of Weight on Adolescent Self-esteem." *Journal of Psychosomatic Research* 38 (1994): 547.

Sayegh, R., I. Schiff, J. Wurtman, et al. "The Effect of a Carbohydrate-Rich Beverage on Mood, Appetite, and Cognitive Function in

Women with Premenstrual Syndrome." *Obstetrics and Gynecology* 86 (1995): 520.

Snider, B. L., and D. F. Dieteman. "Pyridoxine Therapy for Premenstrual Acne Flare." *Archives of Dermatology* 110 (1974): 130–31.

Sonenstein, F. L., L. Ku, L. D. Lindberg, et al. "Changes in Sexual Behavior and Condom Use Among Teenaged Males: 1988 to 1995." *American Journal of Public Health* 88 (1998): 956.

Stead, R. J., S. F. Grimmer, S. M. Rogers, et al. "Pharmacokinetics of Contraceptive Steroids in Patients with Cystic Fibrosis." *Thorax* 42 (1987): 59.

Steel, J. M., and L. J. P. Duncan. "Serious Complications of Oral Contraception in Insulin-Dependent Diabetics." *Contraception* 17 (1978): 291.

Tanner, M., and P. B. Eveleth. "Variability Between Populations in Growth and Development at Puberty." In *Puberty: Biologic and Psychosocial Components,* edited by S. R. Berebberg, pp. 256–73. Leiden: H. E. Stenfert Kroese, 1975.

Troiano, R. P., K. M. Flegal, R. J. Kuczmarski, S. M. Campbell, and C. L. Johnson. "Overweight Prevalence and Trends for Children and Adolescents: The National Health and Nutrition Examination Surveys, 1963 to 1991." *Archives of Pediatric Adolescent Medicine* 149 (1995): 1085–91.

Vignolo, M., A. Naselli, E. Di Battista, et al. "Growth and Development in Simple Obesity." *European Journal of Pediatrics* 147 (1988): 242–44.

Williamson, D. F., and E. R. Pamuk. "The Association Between Weight Loss and Increased Longevity: A Review of the Evidence." *Annals of Internal Medicine* 119 (1993): 731.

Wu, T., P. Mendola, and G. M. Buck. "Ethnic Differences in the Presence of Secondary Sex Characteristics and Menarche Among U.S. Girls: The Third National Health and Nutrition Examination Survey, 1988–1994." *Pediatrics* 110 (2002): 752–57.

Zimmerman, P. A., G. L. Francis, and M. Poth. "Hormone-Containing Cosmetics May Cause Signs of Early Sexual Development." *Military Medicine* 160 (1995): 628–30.

INTERNET SOURCES OF INFORMATION

American Dietetic Association. Available at www.eatright.org.

National Institutes of Health. "Nutrition and Your Health: Dietary Guidelines for Americans." Available at www.health.gov/dietary guidelines.

National Institutes of Health, National Institute of Diabetes and Digestive and Kidney Diseases. "Choosing a Safe and Successful Weight-Loss Program." Available at www.niddk.nih.gov/health/nutrit/pubs/choose.htm.

National Institutes of Health. Weight-control Information Network (WIN). "Weight Loss and Control." Available at www.niddk.nih.gov/health/nutrit/nutrit.htm.

Erika Schwartz, M.D.: www.drerika.com.

Index